State, Society and Health in Nepal

This book focuses on health, healing and health care in Nepal. It presents an intriguing picture: the interplay between the natural processes that cause ill health or diseases and the socio-cultural processes through which people try to understand and cope with them. The work places medical tradition, health politics, gender and health, and pharmaceutical business within the wider politico-economic milieu of Nepal. It also describes the establishment of medical anthropology as an academic discipline, and its relevance for understanding the country's specific health problems, health care traditions, and health policies.

Combining scientific research with practical experiences, the book will serve as a unique resource, especially for health workers, policymakers, and teachers and students in medical schools, those in public health, social medicine, health care, governance and political studies, sociology and social anthropology, and Nepal and South Asian studies.

Madhusudan Subedi is Professor at the Department of Sociology, Tribhuvan University, Nepal where he teaches sociology of health, ageing and disability, and public policy. He was previously Professor at the Department of Community Health Sciences, Patan Academy of Health Sciences (PAHS) and contributed to the development of its curriculum. A medical anthropologist/sociologist by training, he obtained a Master's degree in Sociology from Tribhuvan University and a Master of Philosophy in Medical Anthropology from the University of Bergen, Norway. For almost 20 years he has taught students of medicine, public health, and social sciences. He has conducted extensive research on health issues among people in rural areas of Nepal, and has written and co-authored three books and published more than 30 articles.

Nepal and Himalayan Studies

For a full list of titles in this series, please visit www.routledge.com/Nepal-and-Himalayan-Studies/book-series/NHS

This series brings the larger Nepal and the Himalayan region to the center stage of academic analysis and explores critical questions that confront the region, ranging from society, culture and politics to economy and ecology. The books in the series examine key themes concerning religion, ethnicity, language, identity, history, tradition, community, polity, democracy, as well as emerging issues regarding environment and development of this unique region.

Nepali Diaspora in a Globalised Era
Edited by Tanka B. Subba and A. C. Sinha

Goddesses of Kathmandu Valley
Grace, Rage, Knowledge
Arun Gupto

The Himalayas and India – China Relations
Devendra Nath Panigrahi

Democratisation in the Himalayas
Interests, Conflicts and Negotiations
Edited by Vibha Arora and N. Jayaram

Sex Work in Nepal
The Making and Unmaking of a Category
Lisa Caviglia

State, Society and Health in Nepal
Madhusudan Subedi

State, Society and Health in Nepal

Madhusudan Subedi
With a Foreword by Marit Bakke

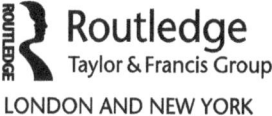

Routledge
Taylor & Francis Group

LONDON AND NEW YORK

First published 2018 by Routledge

2 Park Square, Milton Park, Abingdon, Oxon, OX14 4RN
605 Third Avenue, New York, NY 10017

Routledge is an imprint of the Taylor & Francis Group, an informa business

First issued in paperback 2020

British Library Cataloguing-in-Publication Data
A catalogue record for this book is available from the British Library

Library of Congress Cataloging-in-Publication Data
A catalog record has been requested for this book

ISBN: 978-1-138-55356-9 (hbk)
ISBN: 978-0-367-73533-3 (pbk)

Typeset in Sabon
by Apex CoVantage, LLC

To my mother, Deva Subedi

Contents

Illustrations

Tables

Figure

Foreword

In the fall of 1999 I stayed at the Bergen House in Lalitpur to collect material for a Master's course in 'Communication and Development' at the University of Bergen in Norway. For several years the University of Bergen had rented the building as a base for Norwegian and Nepalese students, teachers, and researchers. When I mentioned the purpose of my stay to Professor Gunnar Haaland, a Norwegian anthropologist who played a major role in establishing this wonderful meeting place, he promptly said: "You must meet Madhu." I met Madhu, and ever since that first meeting we have been colleagues and friends. Unfortunately, the Bergen House closed some years later.

Madhusudan Subedi obtained a Master of Philosophy degree in Social Anthropology at the University of Bergen in 2000, focusing on Human Ecology and Medical Anthropology. He returned to his home country, wanting to establish medical anthropology as an academic discipline in Nepal. There he started as a teacher and researcher at the Central Department of Sociology and Anthropology, Tribhuvan University. Additional teaching at the Institute of Medicine, Tribhuvan University, and at Kathmandu University Medical School (KUMS) gave him a wider exposure in the field. Madhusudan Subedi was among the founding faculty at PAHS, working particularly to develop the Community Health curriculum at the Department of Community Health Sciences. Subedi joined the faculty at PAHS School of Medicine in August 2010 as an Associate Professor and served as Professor from March 2014 to July 2015.

During my visits to Nepal after 1999, Madhusudan Subedi told me about his involvement in creating a unique medical school in that country, first at KUMS, then at Patan Hospital. Dr Arjun Karki was chairing this project, from 2004 assisted by an International Advisory Board (IAB). In April 2006, years of political unrest in Nepal culminated in general strikes, mass demonstrations, and curfews; the monarchy was on the brink of collapse. Despite the challenges for people's everyday life, Dr Karki came to call on me at my hotel in Thamel, and I realized that Madhusudan Subedi had told him about my academic concern for social conditions in Nepal, particularly within the health sector. Dr Karki invited me to join the PAHS International Advisory Board as its only social scientist. It was an offer I could not refuse; the position would enrich my relationship with Nepal, enabling me to contribute my own experiences gained from teaching 'Communication and Development' at the University of Bergen and, not least, from having observed my father's practice as a community medical doctor in Norway. Attending the annual IAB meetings, and collaborating with Madhusudan Subedi and the Community Health Science Group in particular, turned out to be most rewarding. How much I learned about Nepal, its people, and its social conditions! The work culminated with success: in 2010, the first batch of 60 students was admitted to PAHS, and six years later, I congratulated 56 of them on obtaining their license to practice as medical doctors.

Cultural policy and communication have been the major interests during my academic career. Whenever I visited Nepal, I bought books and talked with people about cultural issues, particularly about Nepal's rich cultural heritage. At some point, Madhusudan Subedi and I decided to combine our specialties in an article, he with knowledge of medical anthropology and conditions in Nepal, I with my concern for the crucial role of culture in making communication relevant and effective. The result of our partnership was 'Communication Aspects in Health Care Work in Nepal' – one of the chapters in this book.

Since we first met in 1999, Madhusudan Subedi has been a prolific author of articles on medical anthropology and social conditions in Nepal, addressing issues at the individual and national level. The overall purpose of his academic work has been to provide information and reflections that can improve health care for the population in Nepal, the poor and marginalized in particular.

Textbooks on medical anthropology abound, several of them including some information also about Nepal. But at last, here is a book on social and cultural aspects of health in Nepal only. Most of the chapters have been published previously in Nepalese journals, but they have been thoroughly revised and updated for this publication. By bringing them together, this book offers health workers, health policymakers, and students as well as teachers in medical schools a unique source for obtaining a deeper understanding of the health sector in Nepal.

The first chapter presents an overview of research traditions within medical anthropology. It firmly identifies pluralism as the common theme throughout the book; pluralism in theoretical approaches to and research on health conditions, and in people's and health caretakers' perceptions of causes for illnesses and their cure. Several of the book's chapters illustrate empirically the relevance of pluralism in medical anthropology.

Chapters 2 and 3 look at the options for people who seek help for health matters. These options depend on the variety of healer choices available: a shaman, an Ayurvedic healer, or a doctor trained in western medicine. On the other hand, the options depend on people's perceptions of why they have become sick and what the best treatment is.

The next two chapters focus on indigenous knowledge. Chapter 4 describes traditional health care practices, while Chapter 5 focuses on people's classification of different types of food and how this may affect good health and illnesses. The articles are based on Subedi's observations and interviews in a village in the outskirts of Kathmandu. It is an excellent illustration of the complex set of values and perceptions that health care workers must be prepared for when meeting patients.

In rural areas, many male members of the household are migrant workers, leaving the women behind to till the land, and carry fodder to the animals and wood to the stoves. This is hard work, quite often resulting in the women developing different degrees of uterine prolapse. Chapter 6 presents results from Subedi's observations and interviews during mobile camps in Western Nepal.

Measures for prevention and treatment are equally important elements in any country's health system – many health care workers even put prevention first. Chapter 7 describes the crucial role of communication for obtaining good results in both prevention and treatment. When people know about causes (nutrition, strenuous work, abuse, etc.) for different illnesses, they are better able to take care of their own bodies and health conditions. And when they get sick, people should have information about how they can be treated. On the other hand, health care workers need to know about the potential patients' perception of why they get ill and whom they trust to give the best treatment. Such knowledge is useful for developing communication strategies to reach specific groups. The chapter also illustrates that words matter: different ethnic groups use different words for the same health problem, in this case, acute respiratory infections and illnesses.

To cope with specific health issues requires relevant and correct information. Chapter 8 focuses on disability; first, there is a discussion of the criteria for being defined as a disabled person, then the chapter describes two methods – census and survey – for measuring the prevalence of disabilities. Disability is usually linked to a person's ability to cope with everyday chores. Generally, the survey method includes more disability elements than the census method, the result being that surveys tend to report higher disability rates than censuses. The chapter demonstrates this significant difference with statistics from countries in Europe, Asia, South-America, Africa, and Asia. A special section presents the situation for disabled persons in Nepal.

Several of the chapters show that people seek different types of treatment: shamanistic, Ayurvedic, Homeopathic, Acupuncture, and Allopathic or 'western medicine'. Pharmaceuticals play a major role, usually a positive one, in western medicine. In Chapter 9, Subedi presents a critical overview of the pharmaceutical industry in Nepal. Is it driven by innovation and good practice or is its focus on making money? Experimental production of drugs in Nepal started in 1968, while the country's pharmaceutical industry developed rapidly during the 1980s. Today, foreign, primarily Indian, companies dominate Nepal's domestic pharmaceuticals market. The chapter describes the initiatives that the Government of Nepal has taken to regulate this industry, partly by developing guidelines for the ethical promotion of medicine. Due to actual and potential conflicts of interest between the many national and international stakeholders, it has been difficult to obtain transparency and accountability within this industry, and to secure people's consumer rights.

The final chapter focuses on policy issues that emerge from the information, empirical data, and reflections that have been presented in the book's nine previous chapters. It makes clear the necessity of seeing health matters within a broader context of values, indigenous knowledge, individual and national resources, and the relationships to institutions – not only medical – at the local, regional, and national level in Nepal, and within an international context. This chapter offers comments and criticism of the government's health policies until now, but it also suggests how to improve them.

It has been a pleasure to be involved in preparing this essay collection. It contributes to fulfill the goal for policymaking and practical work expressed in the 1978 Alma Ata Declaration: "To protect and promote health of all the people of the world."

Marit Bakke
Professor Emerita, University of Bergen, Norway

Preface

After completing my MA degree in Sociology from Central Department of Sociology and Anthropology, Tribhuvan University (TU), Nepal, I had an opportunity to teach medical and public health students at the Institute of Medicine, Maharajganj, Tribhuvan University, Nepal. I had no previous experience from teaching medical sociology and medical anthropology, and it was a tough task to give appropriate examples. This opportunity was my 'eye-opening' to be engaged with these disciplines and to become aware of their relevance for positive social development in Nepal. I spent many hours in the library, read books and journals related to thematic subjects. I realized that Medical Sociology and Medical Anthropology were established subjects in the USA and in many European Countries, and in Nepal these subjects were in an infancy state. Professor Mathura Prasad Shrestha, Professor Hemang Dixit, and Professor Yogengra Bhakta Pradhananga, though they were from medicine and a public health background, had wider population health knowledge and a critical understanding of the medical sciences. I used to interact with them on Nepal's population health problems, health inequality, and issues related to 'private profit and common costs practices', healer-patient interaction and communication gaps, health politics, culturally appropriate health policies and programs, and the role of social sciences in medicine. Such discussions further inspired me to learn more about medical and population health perspectives.

In 1998, I received a scholarship from the Norwegian government to pursue a Master of Philosophy in Social Anthropology at the University of Bergen, Norway. There were many books and relevant journals in the university library from which I advanced my learning in medical anthropology and social medicine. Some of the chapters in this book were first written as part of my thesis for which credit goes to Professor Gunnar Haaland who helped me to develop critical social science lenses. His guidance, patience, and genuine criticism helped me to think critically and write something new in the field of social medicine and medical anthropology. Professor Marit Bakke, whom I met in the Bergen House in Lalitpur in December 1999, has always encouraged my academic work and writing. Her constructive feedback and suggestions have been a blessing and inspired me to think, write, and publish academic articles. She accepted my request to collaborate in revising several of my previously published articles for this book. Chapter 7 of this book, 'Communication Aspects in Health Care Work in Nepal', is also co-authored with her. Without her encouragement and dedicated support this book would not have been in the present form. Thank you, Professor Bakke, you have given me power to focus on topics closest to our lives and concerns for population health issues globally and locally.

I took some courses from the Centre for International Health, University of Bergen, Norway in 1999 and 2000. Courses offered by Kris Heggenhougen, Professor of Medical Anthropology at Boston University, who had a wide international experience in the UK, Tanzania, and Norway, provided me a great opportunity to learn social medicine and population health perspectives, and qualitative health research.

The Central Department of Sociology and Anthropology (CDSA), Tribhuvan University has been an inspiring place for me to learn from the faculty and the students, and to share my own ideas, mostly, with the students. I was attached with the CDSA during my study and, since 1996, as a faculty member. At the CDSA, I have academically benefitted from Professor Chaitanya Mishra, Professor Ganesh Man Gurung, and Professor Om Gurung. They have inspired me all the way from my student life at CDSA until today.

For almost 20 years I have been teaching medical, public health, and social sciences students. During and after the classes, students have come and shared their experiences. I feel very comfortable to share my research-based knowledge and to inspire them to explore experiences from their own community and surroundings. During five years as a faculty at the PAHS I learned many things from the young medical students during interactions in the classroom and during field visits in various villages in the Makwanpur District as part of the Community Based Learning and Education (CBLE) program. We used to highlight the saying, "If you hear it, you forget it. If you see it, you remember it. If you do it, you know it." Knowing something means understanding the real scenario of the community and people's day-to-day life related to health. Such personal experiences not only helped the students but also the young faculty. PAHS students used to collect and analyze information at the community level, something that cannot be learned from classroom study alone. I tried to promote health humanities as a means to make better medical doctors. I personally believe that the arts, literature, drama, music, poems, songs, etc. express human creativity, reflecting human joy and sorrow. While in the community, I always encouraged my students to think of themselves as intellectually and morally superior to other medical students who did not have adequate community interaction and exposure. I thank Professor Arjun Karki, the architect and founding Vice Chancellor of PAHS, for inviting me from the initial planning phase of this unique medical school.

The students at CDSA whom I taught courses in 'Culture, Society and Health', 'Sociology of Health', and 'Sociology of Ageing and Disability' have inspired me to publish this book. Some of them are now teaching in public health, nursing, and medical colleges within and outside the Kathmandu Valley. I thank CDSA, TU for providing me the conducive platform and environment to teach, to conduct research, to get involved in public issues, and to publish articles.

In my opinion, a small number of sociologists and anthropologists engaged in the medical and public health institutions do not reflect our potential contribution to the field. A strong coordination is required among the scholars who are engaged in teaching in various universities and colleges, and who are doing health research in Nepal. International academic linkages and collaboration is another aspect for creating greater awareness of these issues. Such collaboration helps critical thinking, writing, and dissemination of the findings to wider audiences. Knowledge about health and disease is not always sufficient to bring about change. We should advocate that health governance focus on equity and social justice, and that health educators share critical ideas, knowledge, attitudes, and feelings.

The book's ten chapters were written over a period of 15 years. In publishing this collection I trust that most of the articles are still relevant for major issues today: health care pluralism, indigenous practices, women and health, health communication and development, disability and methodological challenges, the pharmaceutical industry, health politics, etc. These are some of the key themes around which our social and personal lives are interlinked.

Pratyoush Onta, Seira Tamang, Lok Ranjan Parajuli, and Devendra Uprety at Martin Chautari have always encouraged me to publish a collection of articles. My wife Mina, my daughter Prativa, currently pursuing a medical education, and my son Pratik, have always, despite their own hard work, been encouraging and caretaking so I could accomplish my work.

Finally, I would like to appreciate Man Bahadur Khattri, Editor-in-Chief of the *Dhaulagiri Journal of Sociology and Anthropology*, and Department Head of Sociology, and Editors of *Manav Samaj* and *Vegetation and Society*, for granting me permission to publish articles that originally appeared in their respective journals, but that have been revised for this book.

Acknowledgments

The essays collected in this book have previously appeared in the following publications. They have been revised and updated for this book.

Chapter 2: 'Healer Choice in Medically Pluralistic Cultural Settings: An Overview of Nepali Medical Pluralism', *Occasional Papers in Sociology and Anthropology*, 8: 130–158, 2003.

Chapter 3: 'Illness Causation and Interpretation in a Newar Town', *Dhaulagiri Journal of Sociology and Anthropology*, 5: 101–120, 2011.

Chapter 4: 'Indigenous Knowledge and Health Development in Nepal: An Anthropological Inquiry', *Manav Samaj*, 1: 135–151, 2004.

Chapter 5: 'Explanatory Models of Food, Health and Illness Ideology in Newar Town of Kirtipur', in R. P. Chaudhary, B. Subedi, T. Aase and O. Vetas (eds.) *Vegetation and Society*, pp. 228–239. (Kathmandu: Tribhuvan University, Kathmandu and University of Bergen, Norway, 2002).

Chapter 6: 'Uterine Prolapse, Mobile Health Camp Approach and Body Politics in Nepal', *Dhaulagiri Journal of Sociology and Anthropology*, 4: 21–40, 2010.

Chapter 7: 'Communication Aspects in Health Care Work in Nepal', *Dhaulagiri Journal of Sociology and Anthropology*, 2: 65–100, 2008.

Chapter 8: 'Challenges to Measure and Compare Disability: A Methodological Concern', *Dhaulagiri Journal of Sociology and Anthropology*, 6: 1–24, 2012.

Chapter 9: 'Trade in Health Service: Unfair Competition of Pharmaceutical Products in Nepal', *Dhaulagiri Journal of Sociology and Anthropology*, 3: 123–140, 2009.

1   Traditions in research on society, culture, and health in Nepal

While health, illness, and the practice of medicine are ancient, and all societies have one or several types of healers, biomedicine is a relatively recent phenomenon. Health and illness are variable and people across different cultures and history perceive, interpret, and seek help in different ways. In a market economy, the dominant ways for understanding health and illness is the biomedical model that focuses on curative aspects of health care. An efficient way of making people healthy, however, is to promote healthy behavior by exploring social and cultural aspects of health and illness, determinants of health and the factors affecting people's health, and the way they understand and deal with their own health and illness. It is well known that certain social factors like income, education, occupation, and gender are strongly related to people's health and ill health. Social scientists argue that many causes of health and illness can only be understood from the study of the social, cultural, and the historical surroundings of the people under study. Such surroundings vary from place to place and time to time (Kiefer 2007).

Though Marx and Engels wrote about the health and illness of the laboring population and were concerned with health and illness in relation to living and working conditions, their work did not lead to any development in the sociology of health and illness. Talcott Parsons was the first sociologist who emphasized medicine as a social institution and drew attention to illness as deviance and to the importance of the role of the sick as a mechanism for social control, to the threat that illness constitutes for a society and to the importance, therefore, of the social mechanism. The expansion of medical care to a mass population, with its many problems related to the social organization of intrinsic social interests and technical advances, have added to the range of socio-ethical problems.

Sociology of health has drawn on perspectives and theories from the core sociology ranging from functionalism, interactionism, Marxism, feminism, and post-modernism. The influence of different perspectives varies not just across time, but also between countries.

Social scientists are concerned with social and cultural as opposed to biological factors when explaining diseases. They focus on the etiology of diseases and illness, health seeking behavior, access to and the delivery of health services, consequences of disasters and disability, and ethical, political, and organizational issues in relation to health. Health and illness are shaped and experienced in the light of global, historical, and political forces (Cockerham 2004). The rapid pace of social change – migration, urbanization, and technological advances in medicine – has created new problems in the provision of health care to large sectors of the population. Such conditions and situations not only cause illness, but they also help prevent it. The role of social scientists is to advance thinking and analyzing within a broader framework and to also link micro level events and activities to macro level social issues.

The Alma Ata Conference (1978) strongly reaffirmed that health is a fundamental human right and that the attainment of the highest possible level of health is a most important worldwide social goal that requires action by many other social and economic sectors in addition to the health sector. The Ottawa Charter for the Health Promotion (1986) emphasized that health promotion is the process of enabling people to increase control over, and to improve, their health. This Charter stated that the fundamental conditions and resources for health are these: peace, shelter, education, food, income, a stable ecosystem, sustainable resources, and social justice and equity.

Social and cultural contexts of health are the main focus of 'medical sociology' and 'medical anthropology', sometimes referred to as 'sociology of health' and 'anthropology of health'. I feel it more appropriate to say 'sociology of health' and 'anthropology of health' instead of the more commonly used terms 'medical sociology' and 'medical anthropology'. Both disciplines provide analytical frameworks for understanding the social and cultural context of health, illness, and health care. Medical anthropology focuses more on the cultural context of health, illness, and health care, while medical sociology focuses on the social context. Politics and economics are often of particular interest in medical sociology and medical anthropology because they tend to have tremendous effect on culture and social structures. Different socio-economic groups, for example, often search and use significantly different levels of health care. Inequalities in wealth result in inequalities in health care. The ultimate aims of these disciplines, in my opinion, are to contribute useful and critical knowledge to promote human wellness, to reduce suffering, to improve the treatment of disease, and to meet the urgent practical and moral challenges in complex societies.

The social and cultural context of health research traditions

Understanding the social and cultural contexts of health and illnesses is important for theoretical knowledge and for practical work to change behavior. The ways in which beliefs and behaviors among the population influence the origin of diseases are significant for their health. Such issues can be studied through large-scale quantitative studies among groups of people, as in epidemiological investigations of the distribution of diseases, but also through qualitative investigation of the patterns of health beliefs and behaviors. Qualitative research often uncovers the reasons why particular patterns of illness persist or change.

Sociology and anthropology open the door to gain knowledge about the causes of ill health or diseases, for instance, the hot-cold balance and harmony of humoral medicine, the Yin-Yang equilibrium philosophy of traditional Chinese medicine, the balance of three humors in Ayurveda, and Allopathy explanations for physical injury or pathological abnormality. One cannot expect a doctor trained in the Ayurvedic tradition to understand a person's illness in the same way as a doctor trained in allopathic medicine. Normal behavior in one culture may be considered abnormal in another and, for instance, being judged as mental illness.

Due to its ethnic, cultural, linguistic, and ecological diversity and easy access to research in a relatively small area of land, Nepal has attracted many anthropologists and sociologists, mostly American and European. Nepal is now fortunate to have a considerable number of books and academic articles covering multifaceted dimensions of the Nepali society and culture (Gurung 1990). A small booklet can be prepared if one wants to prepare a bibliography of 'anthropology of health' and 'sociology of health' in Nepal. Most of the research (about 90 percent) has been done by foreign anthropologists, as part of their doctoral work or other projects focusing on Nepal. My intention is not to highlight some and ignore others. I have chosen some themes[1] to make the presentation of information easier.

Shamanism and spirit possession

Health and illness research in its initial phase in western countries emphasized the understanding of 'other cultures' (Lewis 1971). The main aim of medical anthropology is to contribute to and improve the efficiency of public health campaigns implemented in developing countries. The priority of the local context became especially important when conducting research. For much of the 20th century, the concept of local healing practices attracted the anthropologists. This concept was used to describe health practices among different groups in developing countries with particular emphasis on spiritual healings and ethno-botanical knowledge, focusing on magical practices and religious issues and exploring the role and significance of popular healers and their medicating practices. For them, such healing was a specific cultural feature among some groups of people, distinct from biomedicine.

The spiritual basis of the health system among the mountain and hill people in rural Nepal has attracted many anthropologists. Shamanism, like all medical systems, is subject to individual variation, but the system itself and the therapies the shaman provides are largely based upon faith healing or spiritual healing (Hitchcock 1967; Stablein 1976). The concept of illness within shamanistic practices in Nepal is largely perceived as spiritual in nature and illness is often the result of evil forces or supernatural forces.

Shamanism can be categorized into specific types: *Dhami, Jhankri, Jyotisi, Janne Manchhe, Fukne Manchhe, Jharne Manchhe*, and *Herne Manchhe* – all regarded as mediators between the spiritual world and everyday life among various castes and ethnic groups in Nepal, be it in rural or in urban areas. Healing, fortune telling, and consultation with the spiritual world, ceremonies for the dead and the newly born, spells to remove curses, to change bad luck, or to bring love are all parts of the shaman's repertoire. Performances are dramatic – colorful costumes, drumming, chanting, whirling and dancing and singing of sacred songs (*mantras*) to summon deities or expel spirits.

One of the first seminars in Sociology and Anthropology at the Tribhuvan University was held in 1974, and focused on 'Spirit Possession in Nepal'. The seminar book was published in 1976, John T. Hitchcock and Rex L. Jones (eds.) *Spirit Possession in the Nepal Himalayas*. This book contains 19 articles on lamaist spiritual possession and historical observations by scholars, mostly anthropologists who had worked in Nepal. The social, religious, psychic, and therapeutic aspects of spirit possession are dealt with on a broadly regional and ethnic basis.

Literature on the *Dhamis* and *Jhankris* of Nepal and spiritual healing in general is extensive (see, e.g. Michl 1974; Allen 1976; Hitchcock 1976; Hitchcock and Jones 1976; Jones 1976; Macdonald 1976; Okada 1976; Paul 1976; Reinhard 1976; Winkler 1976; Perters 1979;

Shrestha and Lediard 1980; Coon 1989; Desjarlais 1989; Höfer 1993; Gellner 1994; Maskarinec 1995; Miller 1997; Dietrich 1998; Guneratne 1999; Kristvik 1999). Maskarinec's study, based on extensive fieldwork in a blacksmith community in Western Nepal, enriches the complexity of shamanism by a caste perspective and invites a wider comparison both with other Himalayan and with Siberian forms of ritual healing. Dietrich's book (1998), *Tantric Healing in Kathmandu Valley: A Comparative Study of Hindu and Buddhist Spiritual Healing Tradition in Urban Nepalese Society*, and Miller's book (1997), *Faith Healers in the Himalaya*, are classic anthropological studies of the shamans in Nepal. Miller shows the healers in dramatic action, beginning with their participation in an annual 'pilgrimage for power' to a sacred mountaintop, a scene of magical battles in the past.

Many scholars have carefully selected various Himalayan groups, including Tamang, Rai, Sherpa, Gurung, and others, both for their reputations as experienced healers and for their ability to transmit their knowledge to foreign students. A shaman called *Dhami* in Nepal is considered as a lively mediator between the spiritual world and everyday life. Attacks by spirits – *jangalies, masan, bhut, pret, pisach, naagas* – are believed to be the most common causes of illness. The *Dhami* diagnoses come up with the cure, either by making an offering or by suckling out the offending spirit from the patient's body.

In shamanism, illness is caused by malevolent forces, jealousy, an evil eye, or spirit possession. They will prevent illness through the use of amulets or incantations and they will heal illness through the use of exorcism and other rites. According to Vedic astrology, illness is caused by *karma* and the will of the gods. Illnesses can be diagnosed through astrological readings based upon planetary forces and movements and these can be determined through horoscope readings and palm and forehead readings (Dougherty 1986; Subedi 2001). After an astrologer has determined the problem they must determine what will help the patient. Illness is karmic or destined, and an astrologer can learn about your illness through your astrological chart. One can do one or any of the following depending on the illness: performing fire rituals, charitable acts, fasting, giving to the poor, or wearing special amulets. Many scholars have focused on the circumstances of spiritual possessions, on the social, political, and cultural implications of possessions, and on the impact of health on people's lives. They have highlighted, in detail, local social representation and stereotypes.

Nepali scholars have criticized foreign scholars that have tended to focus on shamanistic traditions in Nepal. Mishra (1984), for example, said that there has been too much emphasis on the ideological-spiritual aspect of ethnic groups' traditional healing practices instead of focusing on actual day-to-day problems like poverty, inequality, and marginalization; how can research in sociology and anthropology be justified when the basic problems facing us at large relate to food and clothing? Fisher (1987), however, remarked that health conditions cannot be improved until local healing practices are well understood. Most of the foreign medical anthropologists have tended to concentrate on those aspects of life that seem to be particular, conspicuous, and unique from the western point of view.

The findings from action research conducted by Shrestha and Lediard (1980) showed that the *Dhamis, Jhankris,* and *Janne Manchhe* can play a culturally appreciated and compellingly cost-effective role in the modern health delivery system. The mobilization of these people could tap the indigenous network required to reach and affect the general population with credible and comprehensive messages about health.

Health care pluralism

The dynamics of patient-healer interactions in different cultural settings are a core area of health sociology and anthropology. There are explanatory models of illness and explanatory models of medications due to socio-cultural construction of health, illness, and healing practices. However, the sole objective of the patient is to recover as soon as possible.

Health care pluralism first appeared as a major topic within the anthropological discourse in the 1970s. The key feature of heath care pluralism is the existence and use of more than one health care tradition for the betterment of people's health. Further, the pluralistic structure supports not only the existence of several different, and even competing medical systems, but it also supports the mixing and blending of these systems in both practice and within the beliefs and behaviors of the people who operate within them (Parker 1988). Patients within the pluralistic healing and heath care systems frequently use several different therapies in regard to illness and disease. Different scholars have conducted research on health care pluralism in Nepal (Acharya 1994, 1999; Blustain 1976; Burghart 1984; Devkota 1984; Durkin-Longley 1984; Gartoulla 1998; Pigg 1996; Subedi 1989; Subedi 2001). People in Nepal have been using different health traditions ranging from home-based self-medication and use of different herbals, preference and avoidance of food items, visiting *Jyotishi, Dhami,* and *Jhankri* to Allopathy, Ayurveda, Homeopathy, Naturopathy, Unani, Tibetan Medicine, and Acupuncture.

Devkota (1984) argued that the practice of traditional medicine and its popularity would remain in the foreseeable future. The most important aspect is that perceptions of illnesses and the organization of care for the sick are viewed as a societal matter rather than merely as an individual one. Thus this study reveals the inextricable relationships between society, culture, and disease in any community, linking diagnosis and treatment to culturally specific medical systems.

Subedi (2003) found evidence of health care pluralism, for example, that an individual experiencing chronic joint pain may decide to consult a Western physician, an astrologer, and a shaman, all for the same illness as well as using several different therapies. Patients within medically pluralistic systems will make their personal health care choices based upon the type of illness perceived by the patient. The patients and their family members choose which healers to consult and the kind of therapies to use based upon the nature of their illness and what they perceive to be the problem. Their personal beliefs and the meanings they attribute to their illness will determine both how they understand it and how they will seek to treat it (Stone 1976). Health care pluralism is a result of and affected by larger societal processes, ultimately dictating patient behavior (Subedi et al. 2000).

Ayurveda, feeding, and rituals

Ayurveda is regarded as the old and indigenous medical system in Nepal. It states that the human body is comprised of three elements called *doshas*: air, fire, and water. The body functions when there is a balance between these elements, and a healthy individual will have a standard amount of these elements (Durkin-Longely 1988). A disease is caused when someone has too little or too much of one or all elements. Cameron (1996, 2008, 2009) described the dynamic interplay of Ayurvedic medicine, marginality and Dalit issues, and Gartoulla (1998, 1999) focused on how herbal medicine can be used for treating different health problems.

People in Nepal have for a long time been using various plants to treat specific health problems and it is still a widely practiced form of health care in Nepal (Subedi 2004). Local people have been seeking the underlying causes of health problems and have chosen certain types of herbs to treat them. They also recommended changes in the diet and lifestyle to restore the body's balance during illness and suffering.

Food is vital for the human body to survive. It is associated with the people's socio-cultural, economic, and religious life, thus a socio-cultural approach to the study of food mainly focuses on its ritual and symbolic meaning (Bennett 1976). In Nepal, Lowdin (1985) focused on food rituals and society among the Newars; Subedi (2002) studied food classification among the Newars; and Levine (1988) conducted a study on infant feeding practices in rural Nepal, whereas Gittelsohn (1997) focused on cultural factors, intake of calories, and micronutrient efficiency in rural Nepali households.

Cultural model, schema, and HIV/AIDS

The way people make sense of illness is, in part, culturally determined (Wake 1976). Existing beliefs and presuppositions shared by a community (cultural knowledge) regarding illness play a significant role in shaping an understanding of newly emerging illnesses in any given culture. This cultural knowledge is utilized to 'make sense' of new situations such as the HIV/AIDS epidemic. In this field, the work of Beine (2003) represented an important contribution to the, until then, few anthropological studies of infectious diseases in Nepal by making a long-term study of how local people experienced, understood, and responded to the new and rapidly growing HIV/AIDS epidemic, known only as AIDS, *rog*. His study provided an understanding of the process by which the Nepalese cultural frameworks regarding HIV/AIDS had developed. It also introduced various illness-related cognitive schemata that underlie and inform these cultural frameworks, providing a better understanding of how people incorporate new ideas into established cognitive systems. The study also showed the validity of discourse analysis in linguistic research.

Similarly, Pigg's (2001, 2002a) work on AIDS awareness in Nepal looked at how medical issues link global expertise to local social concerns. She focused on contemporary theories of culture, language, and power; on studies of colonialism and postcolonial social forms; on social analysis of the body, sexuality, medicine, and science; and on questions regarding ethnographic methods and writing. Ghimire (2008) on the other hand, wrote on the broadsheet dailies' coverage of HIV and AIDS issues and themes.

Development discourse and health politics

Many anthropologists have focused on the development discourse in Nepal (Weiner 1989; Thapa 2005; Subedi 2006, 2011b). Stone (1986) examined the primary health care situation in Nepal, its targets and implementation challenges, and in a later study. Stone (1992) focused on cultural influences on community participation in health. Harper (2003) examined the promises of offering capsules to the children in the National Vitamin A Programme. Levitt (1999) highlighted how culturally inappropriate health interventions can be in conflict with traditional ways of managing care in Nepal. Justice (1986) dealt with the bureaucratic structure, culture, and its relationship with the formulation and operation of planning and policies regarding the health sector in Nepal. Her study revolved around some crucial questions such as what kind of information people making plans need and when they need it. This study highlighted that an understanding of the planning process is directly associated with how they affect priorities and points of view and how policies and plans are filtered down through stages of implementation to interact with cultures at the local level. The program that emerges reflects the interactions among the bureaucratic cultures as well as their linkage to the cultures of rural Nepal. Likewise, interaction between international agencies, Nepalese bureaucratic structure and the local culture as a whole, pose different incompatibilities. Foreigners find it difficult to understand the cues and signs in Kathmandu and almost impossible to interpret the complex network of relationships in the district and local administration. Thus, the efforts to deliver health services to rural Nepal encountered not only structural barriers to communication within the Nepali and western bureaucracies but cultural barriers as well (Streefland 1985; Fujikura 2004).

Justice (1986) identified the failure to consider socio-cultural information in planning health care, and argued that there was a chronic gap between policymaking and program implementation. Further, she highlighted that the anthropologists and planners can combine their expertise to make health care programs culturally compatible with the local context. Adams (1998), on the other hand, examined the role of Nepali physicians during the revolutionary changes in 1990. Her study encompassed both the modern political history of Nepal and the role of medicine in a poor, largely rural, Nepal. She found that Nepali doctors were always concerned with developing medical practices that were relevant for Nepali conditions and to take into consideration local conceptions about health. The author emphasized the very fine line between politics and medical truth.

Heydon focused on medicines and travelers (2011a), medicine use historically in rural Nepal (2011b), and medicine and international aid (2009). Dixit (1999) gave a detailed picture of the historical and current state of the health situation in Nepal. Written by a medical doctor, this book begins with a historical analysis and eventually covers contemporary issues such as health rights, primary health care, hospital services, family planning, insurance, diseases, policymaking, medical systems, and medical research. Gautam and Bhattarai (2005) edited a good book about a wide range of issues that enhance an understanding of Nepal's health sector, its policies, plans, and problems.

Medicalization

Medical sociologists and medical anthropologists have also been interested in the expansion of medical control and treatment practices. The concept of medicalization appeared in sociological literature in the 1970s to explain how medical knowledge is applied to behavior that is not evidently medical or biological (Kevin 2002). These sociologists viewed medicalization as a form of social control in which medical authority expanded into the domains of everyday existence, and they rejected medicalization in the name of liberation. Furr (2004) studied the medicalization problem in Nepal.

Mental health and social suffering

There has been a growing acceptance of mental health as an important aspect of health. Mental health is not merely the absence of disease or disorders; it involves self-esteem and ability to maintain meaningful relationships with others (Tausig and Subedi 1997). Mental disorder reflects a socially inappropriate condition that a particular group defines as mental illness and that often includes behaviors that are deemed deviant. It is crucial to understand and explore how the people in specific locations define, interpret, and react with regard to mental health problems of an individual or group. One should examine both interpersonal and institutional aspects of stigma, and give attention to the social processes of rejection or acceptance involved in stigmatization. Issues related to sociological and anthropological understanding of mental health is a relatively new field in Nepal. The mechanisms by which the social environment influences mental health have not been thoroughly studied. Social conditions such as negative life events, ongoing stressful circumstances, demanding social roles, and level of social support are contributing factors for mental health. More research needs to be done to extend our understanding of mental health and illness before developing intervention strategies. Some scholars have focused on mind-body relations, stigma, mental health (Kohrt and Harper 2008), and somatization (Kohrt et al. 2004), but there is much more to be done on mental health in Nepal.

Social suffering takes in the human consequences of war, famine, depression, disease, and human responses to social problems related to political, economic, and institutional power (Ghimire 2009). Social suffering focuses on the mechanisms through which large-scale social forces crystallize into the sharp, hard surfaces of individual suffering in day-to-day life. Structural violence and suffering through the axes of caste, class, gender, ethnicity, religion, and region are some of the areas to be explored in Nepal. Furthermore, the World Health Organization (WHO) now acknowledges that poverty is the world's greatest killer, and the poor are not only more likely to suffer but also more likely to have their suffering silenced.

There are many dimensions of suffering – physical pain, loneliness and isolation, psychological fear, anxiety, depression, despair, and spiritual worries. Desjarlais' *Sensory Biographies* (1992) provided culturally specific events and experiences with great sensitivity, and made them relevant for a broader discussion within anthropology, philosophy, and beyond. Desjarlais' contributions on social suffering focused on healing through images (Desjarlais 1989), body health, on losing the soul (Desjarlais 1992), and on conceptions of death (Desjarlais 2000). His approach, *'kuragraphy'*, prepares us for the complex and often non-linear trajectories of the world (Desjarlais 2003). The Nepalese scholar Kapil Dahal (2010) focused on widowhood, life situations, and suffering during the Maoist war.

Stigma and disability

In disability studies, a person with a disability is seen as having a deficiency and therefore being less able to participate in various work and activities. The social disability model, on the other hand, regards a person with physical or mental impairment as disabled, resulting in society excluding people from participating in ordinary life (Subedi 2012). Social and economic consequences often have been, and are, as important as the physical ones, not only for those affected by the disease but also for their families and communities. Engelbrektsson (2012) highlighted the interplay between disease-specific pathological processes and socio-cultural interpretations and how this explains why leprosy, in spite of the great medical advances, continues to severely challenge the lives of those affected, in many cases even years after being cured, and why the barriers of leprosy-specific self-care are continuously high.

Pharmaceuticals

A less explored but important subject matter of medical sociology and medical anthropology is social and cultural dimensions of the pharmaceuticals. This area has many issues related to society and culture – ranging from World Trade Organization debates on provisions of patent and intellectual property, global pharmaceutical hegemony to subjective experiences of illness and over-the-counter practices. Clinical trials can, and should be, a key research field for anthropologists and sociologists; they can offer distinctive insights into issues of justice within an often shady industry. Outsourcing of clinical trials to lower-income countries like Nepal is a common practice in the global political economy. The poor and uneducated are manipulated, and the testing of new products are not closely monitored by legal authorities. It is important to focus on the recruiting process of researchers and to focus on the patients, the hospitals, and their internal and external dynamics. Recently, some researchers (Subedi 2009; Citrin 2010; Harper et al. 2011; Harper 2014) have focused on the history, dilemmas, ethics, and pharmaceutical regulations in Nepal.

What is missing?

Some thematic areas are yet to be explored by social scientists in general and sociologists and anthropologists in particular. The doctor-patient relationships, including destructive behavior by the patients, relatives, or friends, are important issues in a variety of medical and social settings. Systematic studies on communication of medical information, distortion of understanding, patients' compliance with physicians' instructions, relationship hierarchies, the negotiation of mistakes and trust, etc. are some of the important research areas (Bakke and Subedi 2008). The doctor-patient relationship is influenced by the social setting (e.g. the hospital setting, conflicting interests, structural constraints) and also by the patients' and doctors' internalized expectations (e.g. socialization and social control). Unwanted side effects of medicine due to wrong doses, old and contaminated batches, taking several drugs in a dangerous combination, improperly sterilized syringes, rampant use or underuse of antibiotics and drug resistance, disabling non-disease results from medical treatment and malpractice are on the increase. An understanding of differences of meaning between service providers and service seekers would facilitate new ways of approaching and treating the patients. A comprehensive understanding is important to explore how these complex processes are weaved together.

Outbreak investigations are, generally, primarily designed to identify the sources of unusual diseases or the unusual numbers of cases of particular diseases, as well as to prevent additional cases. Disease outbreaks are newsworthy and a topic of great public concern. Technical experts collect the data, analyze them in sophisticated laboratories, and disseminate the findings. Sociological and anthropological outbreak investigations include disease events and the interpretation of them in the local cultural, social, and economic contexts, as well as comparing such descriptions with people's expectations, their help-seeking behavior, reactions, and interpretations of what is happening. Such information can be used to establish the causes of outbreaks and to analyze social and cultural responses to various interventions. In many cases local disease terminology differ from biomedical ones and care should be taken to understand how local people define disease outbreak. The Government of Nepal, for example, distributes many resources to the regions once an epidemic hits, but does not consider the relevancy of a sociocultural understanding of a disease outbreak in a specific place and time. Sociologists and anthropologists use a number of concepts in order to understand the relationships between the social and cultural context and epidemics, and to explain why particular social, cultural, and environmental conditions are receptive to particular diseases. Thus, they can suggest designing better health intervention.

In Nepal, there has been little focus on the consequences of the neoliberal economic policy and its implication for the poor, on governance and corruption in the health sector, on disability and related policies and implementation challenges, on health inequality, on foreign aid and health politics, and on biomedical hegemony and health humanities. The role of Nepali doctors in the democratic movement (Adams 1998) and the health workers' motivation for joining in the armed conflict (Devkota and Teijlingen 2009, 2010, 2012) have been nicely documented, but the gradual dismantling of the public sector health institutions and the mushrooming of an unregulated private health sector and its impact has not been explored. The situation can be illustrated by the actions of Dr Govinda KC, an Orthopedic Surgeon at the Institute of Medicine (IOM), Tribhuvan University Teaching Hospital, who, by the end of 2017, had fasted close to death thirteen times to stop political interference in the medical sector. Dr KC is recognized widely as a selfless campaigner. His hunger strikes were aimed at fighting corruption fueled by political appointments and vested business interests, and to increase the attention on quality medical education, quality health services, and good health governance.

Conclusion

Health related knowledge is divided into different fields: medical anthropology, social epidemiology, medical sociology, medical geography, medical ecology, medical humanities, bioinformatics, medical demography, etc. Such labeling seems both inevitable and natural but the boundaries between the disciplines are not strict. Integrating knowledge across disciplines involves both communicating ideas across them and recognizing, respecting, and using ideas from multiple disciplines (Trostle 2005). Interdisciplinary exchanges are most productive when researchers work together to define their research questions, objectives, designs, methods, and analyses. Sociologists and anthropologists should actively look for areas where contribution can be made, and to orient teaching, research, and publication to those areas. Sociology and anthropology have been useful in cross-cultural studies of health beliefs and health related behavior, of social and cultural factors related to the utilization of health services, which in turn can be used in both planning and evaluation, on the relationship between behavior and incidence and prevalence of specific diseases, and on the use and acceptance of various types of health practitioners.

Many causes of health and illness can only be understood by studying the social, cultural, and historical surroundings of the people under study (Cameron 2010). Such surroundings vary extremely from place to place and over time. The social perspective on health has powerful political implications, drawing attention to the social processes that lead to poverty and social inequalities, dangerous living and working conditions, poor environmental practices, and the marketing of unhealthy products. It is well known that certain social factors like income, occupation, education, and gender are strongly related to illness rates in almost all societies. A social perspective also draws attention to poor governance, corruption, exploitation, and discrimination. Global opinion has begun to shift towards an increased concern for the health of the poor and for a reduction in health inequalities. Those concerned with health inequalities should focus on reducing the social differences between groups and to improve the conditions among the poor in particular.

In my opinion, the role of health sociologists and anthropologists is to reduce human suffering and to focus on increasing our understanding of the social consequences of illness. Finally, the findings of social science research should be available to people whose lives are touched by the substance of the research. It is the obligation of social scientists to disseminate their works in ways that make it meaningful for appropriate audiences.

Note

1 These tentative themes easily overlap, and one can also categorize the themes differently.

References

Acharya, Bipin Kumar. 1994. "Nature Cure and Indigenous Healing Practices in Nepal: A Medical Anthropological Perspective." In Michael Allen, ed., *The Anthropology of Nepal: Peoples, Problems and Processes*, pp. 234–244. Kathmandu: Mandala Book Point.

Acharya, Bipin Kumar. 1999. "Health Ethics and Choices of Healing: Patient Level Cass from Neuropathetic Clinics." In Ram B. Chhetri and Om Gurung, eds., *Sociology and Anthropology of Nepal: Cultures, Societies, Ecology and Development*, pp. 335–352. Kathmandu: Sociological Anthropological Society of Nepal (SASON).

Adams, Vincanne. 1998. *Doctors for Democracy: Health Professionals in Nepal Revolution*. Cambridge: Cambridge University Press.

Allen, Nicholas J. 1976. "Approaches to Illness in the Nepalese Hills." In Joseph B. Loudon, ed., *Social Anthropology and Medicine*, pp. 500–552. New York, San Francisco and London: Academic Press.

Bakke, Marit and Madhusudan Subedi. 2008. "Communication Aspects in Health Care Work in Nepal." *Dhaulagiri Journal of Sociology and Anthropology* 2: 65–100.

Beine, David K. 2003. *Ensnared by AIDS: Cultural Context of HIV/AIDS in Nepal*. Kathmandu: Mandala Book Point.

Bennett, Lynn. 1976. "Sex and Motherhood among the Brahmin and Chhetris of East Central Nepal." *Contribution to Nepalese Studies* 3: 1–52.

Blustain, Harvey S. 1976. "Levels of Medicine in a Central Village Nepal." *Contribution to Nepalese Studies* 3: 85–105.

Burghart, Richard. 1984. "The Tisyhi Klinik: A Nepalese Medical Center in an Intra-Cultural Field of Relations." *Social Science and Medicine* 18(7): 589–598.

Cameron, Marry M. 1996. "Biodiversity and Medicinal Plants in Nepal: Involving Untouchables in Conservation and Development." *Human Organization* 55(1): 84–92.

Cameron, Marry M. 2008. "Modern Desires, Knowledge Control, and Physician Resistance: Regulating Ayurveda Medicine in Nepal." *Asian Medicine* 4: 86–112.

Cameron, Marry M. 2009. "Untouchable Healing: A Dalit Ayurvedic Doctor from Nepal Suffers His Country's Ills." *Medical Anthropology* 28(3): 235–267.

Cameron, Marry M. 2010. "Feminization and Marginalization? Women Ayurvedic Doctors and Modernizing Health Care in Nepal." *Medical Anthropology Quarterly* 24(1): 42–63.

Citrin, David M. 2010. "The Anatomy of Ephemeral Health Care: 'Health Camps' and Short Term Medical Voluntourism in Remote Nepal." *Studies on Nepali History and Society* (1): 27–72.

Cockerham, William C., ed. 2004. *The Blackwell Companion to Medical Sociology*. Malden: Blackwell Publishing Ltd.

Coon, Ellen. 1989. "Possessing Power: Ajima and Her Medium." *Himalayan Research Bulletin* 9(1): 1–10.

Dahal, Kapil Babu. 2010. "Widowhood, Life Situation and Suffering: A Medical Anthropological Perspective." In Ram B. Chhetri, Tulsi Ram Pandy and Laya

Prasad Uprety, eds., *Anthropology and Sociology of Nepal: Taking Stock of Teaching, Research and Practice*, pp. 305–330. Kirtipur: Central Department of Sociology/Anthropology.

Desjarlais, Robert R. 1989. "Healing through Images: The Magical Flight and Healing Geography of Nepali Shamans." *Ethos* 17(3): 289–307.

Desjarlais, Robert R. 1992. "Yolmo Aesthetics of Body, Health and 'Soul Loss'." *Social Science and Medicine* 34(10): 1105–1117.

Desjarlais, Robert R. 2000. "Echoes a Yalmo Buddhist's Life, in Death." *Cultural Anthropology* 15(2): 260–293.

Desjarlais, Robert R. 2003. *Sensory Biographies, Lives and Deaths among Nepal's Yolmo Buddhists*. Berkeley: University California Press.

Devkota, Bhimsen and Edwin R. van Teijlingen. 2009. "Politician in Apron: Case Study of Rebel Health Services in Nepal." *Asia-Pacific Journal of Public Health* 21(4): 377–384.

Devkota, Bhimsen and Edwin R. van Teijlingen. 2010. "Understanding Effects of Armed Conflict on Health Outcomes: The Case of Nepal." *Conflict and Health* 4(20): 1–23.

Devkota, Bhimsen and Edwin R. van Teijlingen. 2012. "Why Did They Join? Exploring the Motivations of Rebel Health Workers in Nepal." *Journal of Conflictology* 3(1): 18–29.

Devkota, Padam Lal. 1984. "Illness Interpretation and Modes of Treatment in Kirtipur." *Contributions to the Nepalese Studies* 11(2): 11–20.

Dietrich, Angela. 1998. *Tantric Healing in the Kathmandu Valley: A Comparative Study of Hindu and Buddhist Spiritual Healing Traditions in Urban Nepalese Society*. New Delhi: Book Faith India.

Dixit, Hemang. 1999. *The Quest for Health*. Kathmandu: Educational Enterprise (P) Ltd.

Dougherty, Linda. 1986. "Sita and Goddess: A Case Study of the Women Healer in Nepal." *Contribution to the Nepalese Studies* 14(1): 25–36.

Durkin-Longley, Maureen. 1984. "Multiple Therapeutic Uses in Urban Nepal." *Social Science and Medicine* 19(8): 867–872.

Durkin-Longely, Maureen. 1988. "Ayurvedic Treatment for Jaundice in Nepal." *Social Science and Medicine* 27(5): 491–495.

Engelbrektsson, Ulla-Britt. 2012. *Challenged Lives: A Medical Anthropological Study of Leprosy in Nepal*. Gothenburg Studies in Social Anthropology-23. Gothenburg: University of Gothenburg.

Fisher, James. 1987. "'Romanticism' and 'Development' in Nepalese Anthropology." *Occasional Papers in Sociology and Anthropology* 1: 29–42.

Fujikura, Tatsuro. 2004. "Vasectomies and Other Engagements with Modernity: A Reflection on Discourses and Practices of Family Planning in Nepal." *Journal of the Japanese Association for South Asian Studies* 16: 40–71.

Furr, L. Allen. 2004. "Medicalization in Nepal: A Study of the Influence of Westernization on Defining Deviant and Illness in a Developing Country." *International Journal of Comparative Sociology* 45(12): 131–142.

Gartoulla, Ritu Prasad. 1998. *Therapy Pattern of Conventional Medicine and Other Alternative Medication*. Kathmandu: Research Center for Integrated Development (RECID).

Gartoulla, Ritu Prasad. 1999. "Herbal Medicine and Therapy Practices in Nepal." In Ram B. Chhetri and Om Gurung, eds., *Anthropology and Sociology of Nepal: Cultures, Societies, Ecology and Development*, pp. 353–366. Kathmandu: Sociological Anthropological Association of Nepal (SASON).

Gautam, Bhaskar and Anil Bhattarai, eds. 2005. *Health, Society and Politics* (Text in Nepali). Kathmandu: Martin Chautari.

Gellner, David N. 1994. "Priests, Healers, Mediums and Witches: The Context of Possession in the Kathmandu Valley, Nepal." *Man* 29(1): 27–48.

Ghimire, Sachin. 2008. "HIV and AIDS in the Broadsheet Dailies (Text in Nepali)." *Media Addhyan* 3: 99–129.

Ghimire, Sachin. 2009. "The Intersection between Armed Conflict and the Health Service System in Rolpa Nepal: An Ethnographic Description." *War & Social Medicine* 4(3): 139–147.

Gittelsohn, Joel. 1997. "Cultural Factors Caloric Intake and Micronutrient Sufficiency in Rural Nepali Households." *Social Science and Medicine* 44(11): 1739–1749.

Guneratne, Arjun. 1999. "The Shaman and the Priest: Ghosts, Death and Ritual Specialists in Tharu Society." *Himalayan Research Bulletin* 19(2): 9–20.

Gurung, Om. 1990. "Sociology and Anthropology: An Emerging Field of Study in Nepal." *Occasional Papers in Sociology and Anthropology* 2: 4–12.

Harper, Ian. 2003. "Capsular Promise as Public Health: A Critique of Nepali National Vitamin A Programme." *Studies in Nepali History and Society* 7(1): 137–173.

Harper, Ian. 2014. *Development and Public Health in the Himalaya: Reflection on Healing in Contemporary Nepal.* Chennai: Routledge.

Harper, Ian, Nabin Rawal and Madhusudan Subedi. 2011. "Disputing Distribution: Ethics and Pharmaceutical Regulation in Nepal." *Studies in Nepali History and Society* 16(1): 1–39.

Heydon, Susan. 2009. *Modern Medicine and International Aid: Khunde Hospital, Nepal (1966–1998).* New Delhi: Orient BlackSwan.

Heydon, Susan. 2011a. "Medicines, Travelers and the Introduction and Spread of 'Modern' Medicine in the Mt Everest Region of Nepal." *Medical History* 55: 503–521.

Heydon, Susan. 2011b. "Mountains and Medicines: History and Medicines Use in Rural Nepal." *Southern Med Review* 4(1): 4–8.

Hitchcock, John T. 1967. "A Nepalese Shamanism and the Classic Inner Asian Tradition." *History of Religion* 7(2): 149–158.

Hitchcock, John T. 1976. "Aspects of Bhujel Shamanism." In John T. Hitchcock and Rex L. Jones, eds., *Spirit Possession in the Nepal Himalaya*, pp. 165–196. Warminster, UK: Aris and Phillips.

Hitchcock, John T. and Rex L. Jones, eds. 1976. *Spirit Possession in the Nepal Himalaya.* New Delhi: Vikas Publishing Press.

Höfer, András. 1974. "Is Bombo an Ecstatic? Ritual Techniques of Tamang Shamanism." In Christoph von Furer-Haimendrof, ed., *The Anthropology of Nepal*, pp. 168–182. Warminster, UK: Aris and Phillips.

Höfer, András. 1993. "On the Poetics of Healing in Tamang Shamanism." In Bernhard Kölver, ed., *Aspects of Nepalese Traditions*, pp. 155–170. Stuttgart: Steiner.

Jones, Rex L. 1976. "Spirit Possession and Society in Nepal." In John T. Hitchcock and Rex L. Jones, eds., *Spirit Possession in the Nepal Himalaya*, pp. 1–12. New Delhi: Vikas Publishing Press.

Justice, Judith. 1986. *Policies, Plans and People: Culture and Health Development in Nepal*. Berkeley: University of California Press.

Kevin, White. 2002. *An Introduction to Sociology of Health and Illness*. London: Sage Publications.

Kiefer, Christie W. 2007. *Doing Health Anthropology: Research Methods for Community Assessment and Change*. New York: Springer Publishing Company.

Kohrt, B. and Ian Harper. 2008. "Navigating Diagnoses: Understanding Mind-Body Relations, Stigma and Mental Health in Nepal." *Cult Med Psychiatry* 32: 462–491.

Kohrt, B., R. Kunz, J. Baldwin, N. Koirala, V. Sharma and M. Nepal. 2004. "'Somatization' and 'Comorbidity': A Study of Jhum-Jhum and Depression in Rural Nepal." *Ethos* 33(1): 125–147.

Kristvik, Ellen. 1999. *Drums and Syringes: Patients and Healers in Combat against TB Bacilli and Hungry Ghosts in the Hills of Nepal*. Kathmandu: Educational Enterprise (P) Ltd, Mandala Book Point and Ratna Pustak Bhandar.

Levine, Nancy E. 1988. "Women's Work and Infant Feeding: A Case from Rural Nepal." *Ethnology* 27(1): 231–251.

Levitt, Marta J. 1999. "Culturally Appropriate Health Interventions in Conflict with Nepali Management Care." In Ram B. Chhetri and Om P. Gurung, eds., *Anthropology and Sociology of Nepal: Culture, Societies, Ecology and Development*, pp. 309–322. Kathmandu: Sociological Anthropological Society of Nepal (SASON).

Lewis, I. M. 1971. *Ecstatic Religion: A Study of Shamanism and Spirit Possession*. London: Penguin Books.

Lowdin, Per. 1985. *Food Rituals and Society among the Newars*. Uppsala: Uppsala University.

Macdonald, A. W. 1976. "Sorcery in the Nepalese Court of 1853." In John T. Hitchcock and Rex L. Jones, eds., *Spirit Possession in the Nepal Himalaya*, pp. 376–381. New Delhi: Vikas Publishing Press.

Maskarinec, Gregory G. 1995. *The Ruling of the Night: Ethnography of Nepalese Shaman Oral Texts*. Kathmandu: Mandala Book Point.

Michl, Wolf D. 1974. "Shamanism among the Chantel of the Dhaulagiri Zone." In Christoph von Furer-Haimendrof, ed., *Contributions to the Anthropology of Nepal*, pp. 222–231. Warminster, UK: Aris and Phillips.

Miller, Casper J. 1997. *Faith Healers in the Himalaya*. New Delhi: Book Faith India.

Mishra, Chaitanya. 1984. "Social Research in Nepal: A Critique and a Proposal." *Contributions to Nepalese Studies* 11(2): 1–10.

Okada, Ferdinand. 1976. "Notes on Two Shaman-Curers in Kathmandu." *Contributions to Nepalese Studies* 3: 107–112.

Parker, Barbara. 1988. "Ritual Coordination of Medical Pluralism in Highland Nepal: Implications for Policy." *Social Science and Medicine* 27(9): 919–925.

Paul, Robert. 1976. "Some Observation on Sherpa Shamanism." In John T. Hitchcock and Rex L. Jones, eds., *Spirit Possession in the Nepal Himalaya*, pp. 141–151. New Delhi: Vikas Publishing Press.

Perters, Larry G. 1979. "Shamanism and Medicine in Developing Nepal." *Contribution to Nepalese Studies* 6(2): 27–43.

Pigg, Stacy Leigh. 1996. "The Credible and the Credulous: The Questions of 'Villagers' Beliefs' in Nepal." *Cultural Anthropology* 11(2): 160–201.

Pigg, Stacy Leigh. 2001. "Languages of Sex and AIDS in Nepal: Notes on the Social Production of Commensurability." *Cultural Anthropology* 16(4): 481–541.

Pigg, Stacy Leigh. 2002a. "Expecting the Endemic: A Social History of the Representation of Sexual Risk in Nepal." *Feminist Media Studies* 2(1): 97–125.

Pigg, Stacy Leigh. 2002b. "Too Bold, Too Hot: Crossing 'Culture' in AIDS Prevention in Nepal." In Mark Nichter and Margaret Lock, eds., *New Horizons in Medical Anthropology: Essays in Honor of Charles Leslie*, pp. 58–79. London and New York: Routledge.

Pigg, Stacy Leigh and Lineet Pike. 2001. "Knowledge, Attitudes, Beliefs and Practices: The Social Shadow of AIDS and STD Prevention in Nepal." *South Asia* 24: 177–195.

Reinhard, Johan. 1976. "Shamanism among Raji of South West Nepal." In John T. Hitchcock and Rex L. Jones, eds., *Spirit Possession in the Nepal Himalaya*, pp. 263–292. New Delhi: Vikas Publishing Press.

Shrestha, Ramesh M. and Mark Lediard. 1980. *Faith Healers: A Force Change.* Kathmandu: The United Nations Children's Fund (UNICEF).

Stablein, William. 1974. "Mahakala the Neo-Shaman: Master of the Ritual." In John T. Hitchcock and Rex L. Jones, eds., *Spirit Possession in Nepal Himalayas*, pp. 361–375. New Delhi: Vikas Publishing Press.

Stablein, William. 1976. "Tantric Medicine and Ritual Blessings." *The Tibetan Journal: Newark Museum Tibetan Symposium Papers* 1(3/4): 55–69.

Stone, Linda. 1976. "Concept of Illness and Curing in a Central Village Nepal." *Contribution to Nepalese Studies* 3: 55–80.

Stone, Linda. 1986. "Primary Health Care for Whom? Village Perspectives from Nepal." *Social Science and Medicine* 22: 293–302.

Stone, Linda. 1992. "Cultural Influences in Community Participation in Health." *Social Science and Medicine* 35(4): 409–417.

Streefland, Pieter. 1985. "The Frontier of Modern Western Medicine in Nepal." *Social Science and Medicine* 20(11): 1151–1159.

Subedi, Janardan. 1989. "Modern Health Services and Health Care Behavior: A Survey in Kathmandu Nepal." *Journal of Health and Social Behavior* 30: 412–420.

Subedi, Janardan, Sree Subedi, H. Sidky, Robin Singh, J. Blangero and S. William Blangero. 2000. "Health and Health Care in Jiri." *Contributions to Nepalese Studies, the Jirel Issue* (January 2000): 97–104.

Subedi, Madhusudan. 2001. "Development and Under Development of Modern Health Services on Nepal." *Deva Vani* 4(4): 217–224.

Subedi, Madhusudan. 2002. "Explanatory Models of Food, Health and Illness Ideology in Newar Town of Kirtipur." In R. P. Chaudhary, B. Subedi, T. Aase and O. Vetas, eds., *Vegetation and Society*, pp. 228–239. Kathmandu: Tribhuvan University and Bergen, Norway: University of Bergen.

Subedi, Madhusudan. 2003. "Healer Choice in Medically Pluralistic Cultural Settings: An Overview of Nepali Medical Pluralism." *Occasional Papers in Sociology and Anthropology* 8: 128–158.

Subedi, Madhusudan. 2004. "Indigenous Knowledge and Health Development in Nepal: An Anthropological Inquiry." *Manav Samaj* 1: 135–152.

Subedi, Madhusudan. 2006. "Making a Health Public Agenda in Nepal." *Journal of Sociological Anthropological Students Society (SASS)* 1: 73–96.

Subedi, Madhusudan. 2009. "Trade in Health Service: Unfair Competition of Pharmaceutical Products in Nepal." *Dhaulagiri Journal of Sociology and Anthropology* 3: 123–142.

Subedi, Madhusudan. 2011a. "Fallen Womb, Mobile Camp Approach and Social Body in Nepal." *Education and Development* 25: 142–160.

Subedi, Madhusudan. 2011b. "Nepal's Health Sector and Its Sensitiveness (Text in Nepali)." *Civic Health* 1(2): 22–27.

Subedi, Madhusudan. 2012. "Challenges to Measure and Compare Disability: A Methodological Concern." *Dhaulagiri Journal of Sociology and Anthropology* 6: 1–24.

Tausig, Mark and Shree Subedi. 1997. "The Modern Mental Health System in Nepal: Organizational Persistence in the Absence of Legitimating Myths." *Social Science and Medicine* 45: 441–447.

Thapa, Janardan. 2005. "'Scientific' Versus 'Traditional' Cultures: Understanding Cultural Contents for Health 'Development' in Nepal." *Himalayan Journal of Sociology and Anthropology* 2: 18–47.

Trostle, James A. 2005. *Epidemiology and Culture*. Cambridge: Cambridge University Press.

Wake, C. J. 1976. "Health Services and Some Cultural Factors in Urban Nepal." *Contribution to Nepalese Studies* 3: 113–125.

Weiner, Saul J. 1989. "'Source Force' and the Medical Profession." *Social Science and Medicine* 29(5): 669–675.

Winkler, Walter F. 1976. "Spirit Possession in Far Western Nepal." In John T. Hitchcock and Rex L. Jones, eds., *Spirit Possession in Nepal Himalayas*, pp. 244–262. New Delhi: Vikas Publishing Press.

2 Healer choice in medically pluralistic cultural settings

The case of Nepal[1]

Cross-cultural comparisons of health care systems around the world led to the formulation of general models of the relationships between the medical traditions within specific systems. The study of human confrontation with disease and illness, and of people's adaptive arrangements for dealing with ever-present dangers, has become a special branch of anthropology called medical anthropology (Lieban 1977). It is one of the youngest and most dynamic among the various branches of anthropology. It deals with a variety of health related issues, including the etiology of diseases, the preventive measures that members of socio-cultural systems have constructed or devised to prevent the onset of diseases, and the curative measures that they have created in their efforts to eradicate diseases or at least to mitigate its consequences.

The purpose of this chapter is twofold. First, to present some theoretical perspectives on ways to incorporate the 'body' in the 'social reality'. These perspectives have become increasingly relevant with the growth of medical anthropology and its interest in the interface between on the one hand, natural processes that affect the bodies we are 'living in' and, on the other hand, socio-cultural processes in which people understand and cope with their health. Such perspectives enable us to study people's understandings of how their body functions influence health practices, symptom evaluation, and remedial actions. Help may be sought from a number of sources in the patient's social network, including friends, family, traditional healers, and professionals (Christakis et al. 1994; Subedi 2001b).

Our survival as human beings depends on natural processes that involve an interaction between natural processes internal to the body organism, and processes involved in the physical interaction of our bodies with a natural environment. Like for any other species, these processes are subject to 'natural law'. However, in contrast to other species, humans are not endowed with a genetically transmitted repertoire of behaviors which allow a viable interaction in a natural environment. The genetically transmitted repertoires have been softened and weakened to such an extent that human beings neither orient themselves in their world nor communicate with each other without acquiring a great deal of knowledge through learning (Elias 1991). In Geertz's words, "man is an animal suspended in webs of significance he himself has spun" (1973: 5). These webs are clarified through elaborate symbolic exposition.

Without growing up in a context of cultural webs to interpret the interaction between the embodied self and its natural and social environment, the human animal is quite helpless. In other words, humans are situated in an environment that entails both a natural dimension and a culturally constructed one. This 'social environment' is an intrinsic system of interaction between nature and culture, which is created under the specific physical limits that imposes various material constraints upon the human population. As humans we can only experience nature as we culturally construct it, imbue it with meaning, and interact with it in ways that fit within our particular cultural frame of understanding and emotions (Baer et al. 1997: 39).

In this context the most important aspect of this cultural breakthrough is that it implies a conscious ability to see one's embodied self in the perspective of the unavoidability of death. It seems reasonable to assume that the human consciousness of death makes the health of the human body a fundamental concern. This is the general starting point for my description and analysis of the way people in Nepal cope with health in their natural and social environments. Second, this chapter will apply some of these perspectives on health care issues in Nepal.

The impact of the many traditions of medicine in health services remains an area little understood in Nepal. Hence, in determining the factors affecting the different types of health care traditions within a medically pluralistic cultural setting, it is essential to understand how the presence of medical pluralism may be related to or affect the choice and decision to seek different health care services. I argue that the research on illness causality sheds light on health care behavior. Examinations of etiologies entail an exploration of folk epidemiology, factors which lead to vulnerability and susceptibility, as well as on what can be done to avoid the risks.

The chapter is based on my own research of Nepali medical pluralism, and healing and referral processes in the Kathmandu Valley. This has been seen in the context of wider traditions of knowledge and institutional arrangements. Specifically, this study addressed the following questions:

- How do the people in Nepal understand and create meanings on their bodily afflictions?
- How do they relate their health problems with social and natural environments?
- What range of therapeutic traditions is available and practiced in the Kathmandu Valley?
- What are the main causes behind the acceptance of different medical traditions?
- What are the methods used by healers in their healing practices in the Kathmandu Valley?
- How and why are the choices made between and within the various options?

The research was designed to explore the systematic patterns of illness categories among healers and laypersons and their relation to actual behaviors involving those illnesses and help-seeking behaviors in the Kathmandu Valley, given from the point of view of both healers and laypersons. The basic method of data collection was observation along with formal and informal discussions with healers as well as patients. Interviews with different healers took place at the medical shops, health posts, doctor's private clinics (both allopathic medicine and acupuncture therapy), and in the home of local healers, both male and female. I also discussed formally or informally with different people at teashops, and during informal gatherings at the house of different informants.

Several topics were explored simultaneously with different informants. I often followed a sequence of contacts, beginning with local administrators, local health authorities, and the other leaders in the political and administrative hierarchy. The number of conversations and other contacts with these informants varied greatly, depending on their availability, their breadth of information, and willingness to spend many hours with me. My argument is that people's ideas in terms of which they explain and handle illness can be seen as their theory of illness. I wanted to know how patients as well as healers describe their health. For example, what are the locally defined illnesses? What are thought to be the causes and the degree of severity and symptoms? What treatments are sought, and from whom? I also wanted people to talk about their explanations for their state of health; what they identify as important about themselves and their physical or social environments; and what, if anything, they believe can or should be done to protect or enhance their health.

One further interesting venue of research was the attitude of different healers towards the other healing practices and the extent to which the therapy traditions overlap or diverge. My intention was to focus on the interaction of healers and the patients, and how they deal with the different cases of illness they are confronted with.

Theoretical framework

People construct multiple and discrepant worlds by means of different traditions of knowledge available to them. We need to discover how much the different constructions are in fact involved in their actions and interactions (Barth 1993: 271). Following this idea, I have developed my conceptual framework.

Understanding bodily afflictions and explanatory models

Human illness is not only a physical condition but a symbolic one as well. What we experience as health or illness is based on how we judge the relative quality of our physical and psychological condition. The meanings individuals assign to their health status are strongly influenced by their cultural background and experiences (Helman 1996). These culturally based meanings strongly influence the health care choices and decisions they make, their relative confidence in their health care providers and the treatment regime, and even their actual physical responses to health care treatment (Good 1994).

In understanding bodily afflictions, it is useful, in my view, to consider the types of questions that people ask themselves when they feel unwell or when they experience any sudden, unexpected events in their daily lives. My theoretical framework is mostly based on people's understanding of the culturally constructed reality. I argue that the reality can only be fully understood by examining the specific contexts in which an ill person's socio-economic condition and dominant worldviews are patterned. Kleinman (1980) suggested a useful way of looking at the process by which illness is patterned, interpreted, and treated, termed 'Explanatory Models'. This is defined as the notions about an episode of illness and its treatment that are employed by all those engaged in the healing process. Both patients and practitioners hold explanatory models, and they offer explanations of illness and treatment to guide choices among available therapies and therapists, and to cast personal and social meaning on the experience of being ill.

The explanatory model for a particular illness consists of (1) signs and symptoms by which the illness is recognized, (2) presumed causes of illness, (3) recommended therapies, (4) pathophysiology of the illness, and (5) prognosis (Kleinman 1980: 105–7).

As Kleinman pointed out, individuals are likely to have quite vague and indefinite models of explanations for their illnesses, depending on the patients' past experiences, and on their circle of kin and friends (Kleinman 1978). This tendency in research arose, in part, in relation to the growth of cultural pluralism, especially in matters of health and illness (Pelto and Pelto 1996).

Knowledge and concerns

Knowledge in itself is the result of a learning process that is strongly influenced by a number of factors. Once internalized this knowledge becomes belief. Each medical tradition provides a range of beliefs from which people create their reality, the culturally constructed reality. Healers and lay beliefs about health and ill health may differ widely, and these influence the types of conditions that people bring to healers, how they present themselves to the healers, and the types and quality of treatment that they are given. The point is to explore the variation within both lay and professional views, and I have used Barth's (1993: 5) idea of variation to make a sense of people's health seeking behavior:

- There are variations in the definition of illness, and each medical tradition provides unique causes and treatments for a distinctive set of illnesses. Thus over-generalization is perhaps the most serious and frequent weakness of research on health seeking behavior.

- There are variations in the level of 'expertise' within the same medical tradition, and, therefore, no identical, highly rigid pattern of the expertise. Thus, the interpretation given concerning the causes of illness and medicine prescribed varies within the same medical tradition.

These variations are important for better understanding the lives of people, through processes involving their own ideas and activities. The different ways of knowledge transmission generate deep differences in the knowledge's form and scale (Barth 1990: 640). The knowledge that is acquired, retained, and transmitted contains the key to explaining variations.

The arts of impression management

In each medical tradition we can see the interaction as a 'performance', shaped by the environment and audiences, constructed to provide others with 'impressions' that are consonant with the actor's desired goals (Goffman 1959: 17). Each healer promotes the psychological excitement for a realization of a goal. In this way, a healer develops an identity or persona as a function of the interaction with others through an exchange of information that allows for a more specific definition of identity and behavior. There is often a tendency for all types of healers to try to present themselves in such a way as to impress their patients in a socially desirable way. Thus impression management has, in my view, considerable implications for areas of health and healing.

Understanding medical pluralism

Although medical pluralism has been defined differently by different scholars there appears to be a common understanding (Leslie 1980). First, it may mean the coexistence of multiple traditions of medicine, including what are called the folk sector, the popular sector, and the professional sector (Kleinman 1980), offering individuals multiple choices of therapeutic traditions (Minocha 1980; Durkin-Longley 1984).

The *folk sector* encompasses healers of various sorts who function informally and often on a quasi-legal or sometimes, given local laws, an illegal basis. Examples include herbalists, midwives, mediums, and magicians. The *popular sector* consists of health care conducted by ill persons themselves, their families, relatives, social network, and communities. It includes a wide variety of therapies, such as special diets, herbs, exercise, rest, baths, or over-the-counter drugs. Kleinman, conducting research in Taiwan, estimated that 70 percent to 90 percent of the treatment episodes on that island occurred within the popular sector. The *professional sector* encompasses the practitioners and the bureaucracies of both biomedicine and professionalized heterodox medical traditions, such as Ayurvedic and Unani medicine in South Asia, and herbal medicine and acupuncture in the People's Republic of China. Each sector emphasizes the position of patients and healers within different clinical realities. Each type of healers in such a context typically attracts clients from a cross-section of society. Moreover, clients in these settings often try to search around for therapies, making use of more than one of the different therapeutic types available to them during a single illness episode, either simultaneously or in succession (Subedi 1989).

Second, medical pluralism may mean the choices within a particular tradition. An individual has not only a choice between consulting an Ayurvedic practitioner or one practicing Allopathic medicine, but within allopathic medicine, he/she has a choice to go to a particular type of hospital or to a doctor in a private clinic or health post, or to a medicine seller in a village or a town, in a nearby or a distant city. Then there is pluralism in the types of personnel who contribute to the practice of the same medical tradition. Apart from specialists and other registered medical practitioners, there are other personnel, including nurses, technicians, dispensers, and others who not only help the doctors but independently advise and work as medical persons (Justice 1986; Dixit 1999; Kristvik 1999).

Extending the meaning of medical pluralism further, it can be seen as people's conception of disease and illness, their resort to medical practices belonging to different systems, and their responses to other medical dimensions. For instance, people can categorize their illnesses as caused by personal versus natural factors (Foster and Anderson 1978; Foster 1994), and natural versus supernatural factors (Devkota 1984). Villagers resort to indigenous healers for supernatural causes of illness and to allopathic healers for natural causes of illnesses.

To this extended meaning of medical pluralism, one could add the pluralism among the medical practitioners themselves. There is considerable evidence that the general practitioner draws from varied systems in his medical practice. For example, an Ayurvedic practitioner may incorporate in his kit the stethoscope, ophthalmoscope, and other instruments and drugs from modern medicine, and germ and virus theories in his explanatory armory. Similarly, modern medicine practitioners may explain dietary restrictions in terms of the Ayurveda hot-cold dichotomy (Minocha 1980).

Medical pluralism includes both cognitive and social system aspects of healing and treatment traditions. The cognitive dimension relates to a wide range of medical concepts, values, attitudes, and beliefs that serve as guidelines for health related action and practices. Thus, it is easily possible that in one illness episode people have different theories of causality among the various medical traditions. The social system dimension refers to the different economic, institutional, and organizational aspects of treatment and health care delivery. In looking at health care pluralism, wherever it occurs, it is important to examine both the cognitive and the social aspects of various types of health care available to the individual patient.

Medical pluralism in Nepal

The existence of several therapeutic traditions in a single cultural setting is an especially important feature of medical care in the developing world (Leslie 1978). Patients may feel uncertain as to what type of care can cure their illness, leading them to consult different medical therapists. Or they may decide that treatment of a certain illness requires more than one type of assistance. Generally, care is sought from several types of providers and medical traditions concurrently or sequentially. The practitioners of different medical traditions may interact with each other in a variety of ways – at times they borrow the ideas and knowledge from each other, compete with and oppose the other system, they may cooperate with other developing referral systems or they may simply coexist independently of each other (Kleinman 1980; Levitt 1988; Subedi 1989).

The pluralistic character of health and medical systems in almost every society, be it simple or complex, is increasingly recognized (Minocha 1980; Subedi 1988). This pluralism may receive state recognition and patronage, or the state may discourage it or remain neutral to its existence.

Health and healing in Nepal comprise a wide range of medical beliefs, knowledge, and practices. This section describes the several types of practitioners, including medical doctors (specialized in allopathic medicine),[2] health assistants, nurses, dispensing chemists and pharmacists, acupuncture therapists, Tibetan medical practitioners, Ayurvedic[3] practitioners, Unani medical practitioners[4] folk healers, tantric healers, spiritual healers, *Dhami* and *Jhankris* (shamans), herbal doctors, traditional birth attendants, and other practitioners. Informal or even illegal medical traditions are available as numerous alternative therapies. In the application of their medical knowledge, these doctors and healers use different forms of diagnosis, therapy, and medicines. They elaborate, develop, and modify the old traditions and make new ones. Although a certain variation in medical knowledge, specialization, and curing practices is found in almost all societies, in Nepal this variation is pervasive, and it may be the manifestations of cultural pluralism that characterizes many Asian societies.

The state-funded health services in Nepal are also pluralistic in character. There is not only one type of health service in the country, nor is there uniformity among various health services. To name only a few, there are the Police and Army Hospitals that cater particularly to their employees and their family, the Tribhuvan University Teaching Hospital, and other private or public medical college hospitals, mission hospitals, and numerous others. Within the Kathmandu Valley itself it is estimated that there are more than 1,200 government and private medical agencies, missionary- and community-managed hospitals, health centers, health posts, and sub-health posts, and other facilities. Service charges, indoor and outdoor facilities, and specialties are different in each health institution.

In order to understand the health care choices people make when having health problems it is important to recognize the various medical traditions that influence people's decisions. In Nepal, the several medical traditions with their independent classification of illness, theories of disease causality, diagnostic methodologies, practitioners, and treatment therapies present the health seeker with a wide menu of alternatives to choose from. These next sections describe three medical settings and their associated medical traditions, here presented in a simplified version to provide the reader with some sense of the distinctions between them.

Household-based self-medication

Household production of health recognizes that a person's access to and use of various forms of treatment are connected to his or her social power in relation to other household members. Here, a household is examined rather than a family, as a household may be easier to define. A household may include, for example, other relatives living in the same house. Household productions of health examine how household members cooperate and compete for resources in order to restore, maintain, and promote health. Caretakers attend to the patient through examinations, diagnosis, and treatments.

Medical conditions necessitate a variety of changes in a household. Indeed, the full extent of the resources and responsibilities, which need to be negotiated, may not be recognized by outside observers. These include fees for medications, analyses, and examinations; transportation costs; arrangement for accompaniment; and loss of one worker, more likely of two workers, who take care of household chores or provide income from jobs. All these factors, and no doubt more, can influence heath care seeking decisions. Considering the possible impact of the medical condition on the household helps explain why patients may come to the hospital too late for treatment.

As mentioned, a person's access to health care is often influenced by his/her position within the household. One member may receive immediate treatment or the more prestigious treatment, while another member may receive care only if the symptoms are prolonged or may receive less prestigious treatments, such as home remedies. Among the characteristics influencing a person's status within the household are his/her age, gender, marital status, and work status. Due to differences in roles, status, and responsibilities within a household, various members' medical conditions affect the household differently and also their access to treatment differs.

Further, a person's position within the household also influences his/her sick role behavior. Thus, a high status individual or wage earner may receive concern and medical attention over a cough, whereas a lower status individual may have to really moan in order to appear sick enough to receive attention. When an illness strikes, the afflicted person generally does not cope individually – a whole network of supporting social ties are mobilized. The composition of members in this network is of course decided by the structural principles according to which right and obligations as well as emotional involvement tie individuals to each other in enduring groups.

In Nepal, the most important group is the patriarchal household (nuclear or joint). Although there are significant variations among households with regard to social, cultural, and economic 'capital' (Bourdieu 1977), one of their dominant concerns is biological reproduction. Everywhere in Nepal, the household is the key group for socializing the children and providing livelihood for its members, and is, therefore, mobilized when a disease strikes. Important stores of knowledge transmitted within households are brought into play when the health of its members is threatened, particularly children, old people, and the disabled.

Almost all households, at least at the initial stage of an illness, utilize a fairly wide stock of inter-generation transmitted as well as newly acquired knowledge and practices of healing to nurse the ill back to good health. The localized nature of society; the limited access to, and relatively low quality of, public health institutions; and the prohibitive costs of allopathic medicine and modern health services also force most households to rely on home remedies, which span from divination to faith healing and the use of local herbs. Increasingly, they also involve the use of over-the-counter allopathic drugs, which remain almost completely unregulated (NESAC 1998; Subedi 2001b). Using massage, administering herbs, manually removed obstructions, applying heat compresses, and recommending dietary restrictions and prescriptions are the major self-medication practices in Nepal. Generally, medical problems are first treated at the home with some remedies suggested by relatives and neighbors. A specialist is called on only after several attempts have failed.

While access to the health posts or hospitals is easier now than in the past, home-based treatment is still playing an important role in health seeking behavior. For example, the majority of child births in Nepal take place at home rather than in health facilities. The rise and expansion of hospitals and other health institutions for enhancing individually based knowledge can be expected to change the household-based self-medication.

Local indigenous medical traditions

In general, when the home remedy to cure an ill person fails, a larger net of intervening agents is brought in, namely community healers. They may vary among and within religions and ethnic groups, and locally they operate without any government recognition or formal coordination. Their medical traditions and practices may be based on religious beliefs regarding cosmos, ideas about the cultural construction of persons, personal relationships between humans and the environment, and diet. Healers often specialize in particular techniques, and which specialist is consulted depends on the nature of the illness.

In terms of religion, one's health or ill health can be attributed to one's relationship with the spiritual world of anti-gods (demons) and gods (whether one has satisfied or angered them), the relationship between the deeds of one's past lives and one's present life (predestination, fate), and one's deeds according to Hindu and Buddhist scriptures (virtuous or sinful) (Hitchcock and Jones 1976; Miller 1979; Dietrich 1998). In this tradition, one explains illness in terms of *dharma* (religion) or *karma* (fate), prevents illness by following rituals properly, making promises to the gods, giving offerings and doing sacrifices, through prayer, and by following the scripture. Illness is diagnosed and cured by *jyotisis* (astrologers), *guru-purohits* (priests), or monks through prayers and rituals.

The magical, spiritual world affects health and can cause illnesses through the network of angry ghosts (spirits of persons who have died in violent or other unnatural deaths), monster-like *bhut-prets* (spirits), angry gods and anti-gods, and *bokshis* (witch person who can cast evil spells by performing inverted religious rituals). In this tradition, illness is believed to be caused by supernatural attacks (*lagu, lagu-bhagu*) resulting from jealousy (especially in the case of witches) or by having ignored or offended a spirit (Pigg 1989). Attacks can be in the form of possession or some type of physical harm. Specialists who help to diagnose and cure illness brought on by such attacks are commonly referred to as faith healers, including sorcerers (those who can cast and break spells and have the ability to communicate with the spiritual world), shamans (those who go into spiritual possession trances, can perform exorcism and can act on the behalf of spirits), and mediums or *Janne Manchhe* (those who can act as transmitters between the spiritual world and the non-spiritual world).

A study in 1977 estimated the number of various categories of faith healers in Nepal to be between 400,000 and 800,000 (Shrestha and Lediard 1980). With a population of about 13 million this roughly translated to one faith healer for every six households. The number of doctors at the same time was 500, and the number of nurses 334 (Shrestha and Lediard 1980: 34). This figure can be taken as an indication of the legitimacy of the healer tradition. Different research findings (e.g. Okada 1976; Durkin-Longley 1984; Gellner 1994) show that even close to the hospitals in the Kathmandu Valley, traditional healers are many, and in high demand. Diagnosis is done by going into trance, divination, and by inquiring about and observing physical symptoms. Preventing an attack is done through rituals, by providing the individual with an amulet, by being careful not to offend spirits or persons suspected of being witches, by keeping a fire lit, by being cautious of persons seen at night, and by staying away from haunted places. Treatment is done by chanting mantras and shouting at the spirits to leave the person's body, violent exorcisms by which the patient is burned, frightened, and beaten until the spirits flee the patient's body, and by giving offerings and doing sacrifices. The significant role of the local healers has been widely noted in different parts of Nepal (Blustain 1976; Okada 1976; Stone 1976; Wake 1976). The majority of sick persons in the rural area, who eventually visit the allopathic healers, consult the traditional healers first.

Ayurvedic, Homeopathic, and Unani traditions

The Ayurvedic medicine is based on the classic Sanskrit medical tradition of 'Ayurveda' (literally 'science of life'). This tradition of healing has been practiced in South Asia since ancient times (Durkin-Longley 1988). It is based on a well-developed system of physiological characteristics of the ill person, symptoms of illness, and detailed pharmacological knowledge of herbs and their processing techniques.

Within the Ayurvedic medical tradition a person's body is composed of *prakriti* (the female component of the cosmos which forms the body) and three *doshas* (humors) (air, fire, water) that are responsible for all bodily processes. The equilibrium of the *doshas* maintains health and an imbalance results in ill health. In this tradition, diseases or disorders are caused by physiological imbalances resulting from poor food habits, environmental changes, and shock to the system. Diagnosis is done by pulse reading, physical examination, and appraisal of symptoms. Disorders are treated with herbal medicines, diet control, lifestyle control, surgery, meditation, and changing one's environment.

Many Nepalese believe in its efficacy in the long run, that is, as capable of achieving more permanent healing with no harmful side effects.

The Government of Nepal has formally recognized this medical tradition, and there are several government-affiliated Ayurveda institutions. For example, the Institute of Medicine, Tribhuvan University has an Ayurvedic campus in Kathmandu, there is a Department of Ayurveda in the Ministry of Health, and there are also some recognized health centers and pharmacies. Some Ayurvedic practitioners have their own private clinics. Ayurvedic doctors attend medical schools either in Nepal or in India for a degree in Ayurvedic Medicine and Surgery. As early as the mid-1980s it had been estimated that there were 1,500–2,000 Ayurvedic practitioners in Nepal and 113 government Ayurvedic dispensaries (Streefland 1985). Most Ayurvedic healers in Nepal work within the private sphere. There is a policy to provide Ayurvedic services up to the village level and accordingly there is a plan to establish 100 dispensaries, 50 health centers, 3 regional hospitals, 1 training center, and 5 herbal gardens in each development region. Currently, public sector Ayurvedic healing is performed through 2 Ayurvedic hospitals, 14 zonal dispensaries, 50 Ayurvedic health centers, 211 Ayurvedic clinics, and a central drug-manufacturing unit (MoH 2016). However, fewer resources are devoted to them than to Allopathic medicine.

As per the policy of the government to provide health care to all people in an easy and accessible manner, the homeopathic system of medicine is formally recognized in Nepal. Homeopathy was introduced in Nepal as early as 1920 as a natural healing system. Homeopathic healing is largely a private sector initiative and most of them work independently and hardly share their experiences to other professionals. The pharmaceutical companies have little connection with homeopaths. Within the public sector, there is only one homeopathic hospital in Nepal.

The Unani healing tradition, with preventive, promotive, and curative services, has an extremely limited reach. In addition, the Tibetan healing tradition, acupuncture therapy, Japanese healing cults (*Seimeiko*), and Naturopathy are also practiced in selected areas of the country

Allopathic medical tradition

This tradition is based on the germ theory of disease and studies of anatomy and physiology. The worldview that has shaped the allopathic medicine is commonly referred to as the mechanistic paradigm,[5] the characteristic being the separation of the component parts and emphasis on a detailed study of them. According to this tradition, ill health, manifested by various signs and symptoms, results from pathological processes in the body's biochemical function. In this medical tradition, health and normality are defined by reference to certain physical and biochemical parameters, such as weight, height, blood pressure, heart rate, or visual activity. For each measurement there is a numerical range of normal values within which the individuals are assessed as healthy. Above or below these ranges are abnormal conditions.

In this tradition, medical treatment is based on the theory that a disease can be carried from person to person, through the air, through the blood or bodily secretions, or from contact with a septic object or substance. Allopathic medicine was introduced in Nepal at the end of the 19th century when the Bir Hospital was established in Kathmandu, and organized development of allopathic services started in the mid-1950s. This system is formally associated with the public health care system in Nepal through the Ministry of Health and a number of private offices staffed by physicians, public health professionals, nurses, midwives, health assistants, pharmacists, village health workers, and trained volunteers. Diagnoses are made by physical examinations, appraising symptoms, taking blood pressure, doing laboratory tests of blood, urine, and stool, taking the body temperature, and taking X-ray and CAT Scans. Treatments are given through injections, medication, blood transfusion, surgery, electric shock, bed-rest, recommending behavioral or dietary changes, and physiotherapy. Prevention of diseases and illnesses are done through immunizations, health education and promotion, birth control, dietary restrictions, and early examination and screening. Nepali people have a considerable faith in the technology of allopathic medicine, particularly in injections and antibiotics (Gellner 1994). A wide range of allopathic medicine manufactured in India and Nepal are freely available without an authorized person's prescriptions. The people in charge of medical halls and pharmacies lack any formal training and are selling 'prescription only' drugs.

Allopathic medical facilities, pharmaceuticals, and trained personnel, however, are neither reliable nor easily available in rural areas. Almost 50 percent of the country's doctors, the most sophisticated and large private nursing homes and hospitals, trained medical professionals, and the health facilities are concentrated in the Kathmandu Valley. Government-run health services provide care unevenly in the countryside; it is remote and inconvenient for allopathic practitioners (Macfarlane 1994; Pigg 1995). Maintaining a supply of drugs to remote health posts is a constant problem, as is keeping health posts and district hospitals staffed with trained, active practitioners (Justice 1986).

In my view, biomedicine must be seen in the context of the capitalist global system. Some of its particular agents include international health agencies, foundations, and national bilateral aid programs. Most of them are multinational corporations, especially drug firms, medical technology producers and suppliers, polluting and exploiting industrial firms, agribusinesses, commercial baby food suppliers, purveyors of chemical fertilizers and pesticides, and sellers of population control devices. Their activities are supported by a worldwide medical cultural hegemony that also affects activities at the national level (Elling 1981, quoted in Baer et al. 1997). The industry's profit-making orientation caused allopathic medicine to evolve into a capital-intensive endeavor heavily oriented to high technology, the massive use of drugs and the concentration of services in medical complexes. The state legitimizes corporate involvement in the health arena and reinforces it through support for medical training and research (Baer et al. 1997).

There are a number of characteristic tendencies in Nepal's allopathic medical tradition. The first tendency is that the location of medical hospitals and research institutions and allocation of resources are centralized in urban areas. The largest, most prestigious, most specialized, and most money-consuming curative institutions are located in the large urban centers (Streefland 1985; Subedi 2001a). The same applies to the location of institutions where medical knowledge is developed, stored, and taught. It is difficult to find medical schools, libraries, and research centers outside the larger towns. The politicians and administrators who steer and make decisions regarding the country's health policy live and work in Kathmandu, the capital city. Similarly, the drugs to be used are generally manufactured in the urban centers or in rich countries. Nepal's ruling elites collaborate with international agencies, foundations, and bilateral aid programs to determine health policies (Justice 1986). These elites and the agents they deal with often advocate nationalized and preventive medicine, but their actions favor curative rather than preventative health care for themselves and even for the lower social strata in the name of 'medical tourism' or 'medical centers'. This situation clearly shows that the further away people live from the center in physical and/or social distance, the more difficult it becomes to get a good quality and sufficient quantity of medical supplies, facilities, and health workers (Streefland 1985). This holds for remote villages and for urban slums. Although urban health care institutions and medicines are within a reasonable distance for the poor, the costly nature of allopathic medicine plays an important role for not consulting the allopathic medical practitioners.

The second tendency of the allopathic medicine is that, in developing countries like Nepal, allopathic medicine is highly commercial in orientation. Many curative institutions, pharmaceutical companies, and medical equipment industries are privately owned. The goal of many medical practitioners is to work privately and earn more money. Profit-making is an important consideration in the delivery of health care, and the production and sale of drugs and materials. The consequence of such factors is that, broadly speaking, the best services and facilities are available in those places where most people are living and where most wealth is concentrated. For the rural villages it means relatively low numbers of drug sellers and relatively unqualified medical practitioners (Subedi 2001a). On the other hand, the large demand for curative services creates an excellent environment for the activities of unqualified medical practitioners and unlicensed drug sellers.

Interaction between medical traditions

These different medical traditions do not exist as closed cultural systems. Their practitioners interact with one another in a variety of ways, and at times they borrow, compete with, and oppose each other. They may cooperate in moving patients through particular referral systems. Through such interaction there may develop a certain integration of elements of knowledge from different traditions. Other elements in their traditions and practices may remain intact and coexist independently. For example, traditional healers may give modern medicine; faith healers and traditional birth attendants are being trained as village health volunteers and community health leaders; physicians may prefer Ayurvedic medicine for hepatitis; local Ayurvedic healers or herbalists, after being unsuccessful in curing a patient, refer patients to a hospital; whereas spiritual healers or shamans condemn beliefs about ghosts and witches as superstitious. Durkin-Longley (1984), in a study of urban Nepal, showed that specific illnesses ideally are brought to practitioners of one medical traditions: jaundice (*kamal-pitta*) is brought to the Ayurvedic doctor, mental illness to the *Dhami*, *Jhankris*, and *Jharphuke Vaidyas*, and accidents to the modern, allopathic medical practitioners.

Not all systems exist to an equal extent in all parts of Nepal. The local indigenous system exists to a far greater extent in rural areas than either the modern medical or Ayurvedic systems do. However, everywhere in Nepal there is a pluralistic medical setting in which people must make their health care choices.

Factors that have influenced development and acceptance of medical traditions

Different medical traditions in Nepal coexist very well. Each tradition has its own expertise, especially in certain illnesses. In many cases, the question of which specialist to consult depends on the nature of the illness. For example, most of the people seek Ayurvedic *Vaidya* or Kaviraj for jaundice, and *Dhami, Jhankri, Janne Manchhe, Jharphuke Vaidya*, or other local healers for *lagu* or evil spirits. Minor discomfort, wounds, and sores are often treated at the home with foods and herbs; for more serious injuries, hospitals, clinics, or health posts (allopathic healers) are consulted. Except for this, the larger pattern is not a matter of whom one consults when, but whom one consults first and why.

People's actual health behavior when having choices is the outcome of the weighing process where various factors are taken into account. One factor is the perception which villagers have of the health care personnel. For instance, my study (Subedi 2001b) of health seeking behavior in Kirtipur clearly showed that certain healers who belonged to the same village, and thus were related to their clients also as kinsmen, neighbors, or *afno manchhe*, often were more popular than healers from outside the village. Other factors are the cost of treatment compared with what people can afford and to the quality of service they will get. The actual cost of using the services, getting to the services, and the opportunity cost (loss of money which could have been earned instead of seeking help) are also important.

Cultural and historical forces

People's understanding of their bodily affliction and search for cure is one of the most powerful forces in maintaining the continued acceptance of any medical tradition. The members of each cultural group have deep-rooted beliefs that their own tradition must be useful, if not the ideal one, for handling illnesses that occur. Many informants in my study said that healers such as *Jharphuke* or *Janne Manchhe*, not allopathic medical practitioners, could cure illnesses they believed were caused by ancestors, *bokshi, Ajima*, and other types of *lagu*-inflicted illnesses.

Since ill health is defined somewhat differently from culture to culture, and certain diseases are believed to have supernatural causes, including *bhut-pret* and *bokshi*, particular treatment is, therefore, recognized only by its own members. Some culture-bound syndromes, such as *sarko*, *janaikai*, and *bokshi bigar*, play an important role to prolong and reinforce existing medical traditions and their concepts of the universe. This is particularly the case in relation to psychological illnesses. Where the cultural perceptions differ substantially between the sick individual and the therapist, treatment will be extremely difficult. Many of my informants thought that they should try to find different types of healers within as well as across the traditions simultaneously, altering between them or use them sequentially in the hope that one, if not all, would eventually help them to get rid of their illness.

Most of the patients' version of their use of different healers varied according to the nature of the culturally perceived diseases and what they assessed as the best treatment. For instance, patients with constipation, jaundice, or respiratory problems preferred Ayurvedic healers due to long-term beneficial results, whereas allopathic drugs relieved them temporarily. According to them, allopathic remedies were mostly effective on accidental injuries. Likewise, *tantric* healers or *Jharphuke Vaidya* were perceived more effective against *lagu* and *bokshi bigar*. After having consulted a variety of healers with a range of remedial actions, they had obtained experiences that enabled them to feel, perceive and value those healers.

Economic forces

The cost of and access to medical care are equally important factors that influence the choice between medical care traditions. In developing countries like Nepal, where the bulk of people live in poor economic conditions, the cost of medical specialist doctors' fees, pathological tests, and medicines are usually beyond their means. The government expenditure on health is generally low, and health services are beyond the reach of a large number of people living in villages and remote areas. With a minor illness, most people in the Kathmandu Valley seek local healers or buy easily accessible and affordable medicines in over-the-counter shops. Therefore, people often have to depend upon locally available health facilities which are within their geographical and economic reach.

Influence of other medical traditions

If the dominant medical tradition is unable to provide the population with adequate health care, other medical traditions fill the gaps. If a patient uses a variety of remedies but does not recover, he/she tries to find alternative therapies or cures for the disease. People adapt the recommended behavior within a particular medical tradition without knowing much about it. They may, in other words, seek a remedy for the purely pragmatic reason that they perceive it as being effective. For example, some patients learned about acupuncture as an alternative medical treatment, but most of them said that they approached acupuncture clinics as the final attempt before they might die. They had been frustrated with a painful life with chronic sufferings, spent thousands of rupees and visited a number of medical specialists in the country. In the end, many people thought: "why not once experience acupuncture?"

Finally, procedures employed for diagnosis, treatment, or cure by different health care practitioners are closely related to their efficacy. Besides, when healers and patients perceive knowledge and values on physical, mental, or spiritual concerns differently, the healers play a decisive role, whether patients seek them or not. For example, during discussions in my study, patients commented that they preferred kind-hearted, smiling, cheerful, friendly healers who listened to their sufferings. The patients searched for relatively expert, senior, and experienced health professionals who could offer any kind of remedy from which they could recover quickly. If the remedy had harmful side- or after-effects, they would seek other healers they hoped could cure them without such effects.

Concluding remarks

A number of studies in Nepal have shown that persons seek different types of healers based on their perception and beliefs regarding the illness problem, which in turn are influenced and defined by their social surroundings and social network. The most widely prevailing medical tradition in Nepal is faith healing. The fatalistic nature of people plays a distinct role in Nepali society, especially when someone in the family suffers from chronic illness, mental illness, or is not able to have even a single child. Hence faith healers or shamans, such as *Dhami*, *Jhankri*, *Lama*, *Guruwa*, receive wide public acceptance and play a significant role in meeting the health care needs of the villagers. The patients in the hilly regions of Nepal are more likely to contact *Dhamis* and *Jhankris* first before other health care providers.

Most patients in Nepal use home remedies and delay seeking professional help. These remedies included herbs and foods to eat or avoid. If the problem continues, the next resort is a traditional healer. The modern health care services are only sought as a last resort, usually for serious and persistent problems. Research findings also show that patients who do seek treatment at health facilities use both traditional and modern medicine according to their perceived effectiveness.

The point is that treatment decisions in medically pluralistic settings in developing countries like Nepal are complex. The choice of healers is shaped by a wide range of factors, among them perceptions of efficacy, practical considerations (such as distance), symbolic considerations, the perceived cause of the ailment, whether it is viewed as life threatening, and the patient's personal attributes. A variety of research shows that the existence of biomedicine is one among several treatment options and that the presence of alternative sources of health care can significantly affect the choice of health care services. This chapter has showed that anthropological knowledge and research methods have not yet realized their full potential for contributing to contemporary health issues. Thus, in assessing the use of health care services, various factors associated with medical pluralism need to be considered seriously.

Notes

1 A version of this chapter originally appeared as 'Healer Choice in Medically Pluralistic Cultural Settings: An Overview of Nepali Medical Pluralism', *Occasional Papers in Sociology and Anthropology*, 8: 130–158, 2003. Used with permission.

2 I use the term 'allopathy' in a neutral sense. Although, here, I am not going to specify the terminological issues, different writers have used the words like 'cosmopolitan', 'western', 'modern', and 'biomedicine', which is synonymous with *angrezi* (English) system. As Leslie (1976) noted, to call it 'modern medicine' suggests a contrastive relationship to some conservative 'traditional medicine'; to call it 'scientific medicine' suggests that other medical systems are unscientific. Similarly, to call it 'western medicine' is to overlook its use in other parts of the world. However, these different words are used synonymously to refer to the allopathic medicine. Practitioners of this tradition in Nepal are called doctors (physicians and surgeons), health assistants, nurses, assistant nurse midwives, and so on.

3 Ayurveda, literally 'the knowledge of life', refers to the vast body of ancient Hindu literature concerned with health and disease. The traditional practitioners in this tradition are usually called *Kaviraj* and *Vaidya* in Nepal. Similarly, the word *Vaidya* refers to a wide variety of healers. A broad division can be made between those who stick exclusively to Ayurvedic methods and diagnoses, and those who make use of an eclectic mix of Ayurveda, astrology and tantric rituals. The latter are called *jahrphuke Vaidyas*, that is, who use the technique *jharnu* (sweeping) and *phuknu* (blowing). Both Ayurvedic practitioners and ritual healers are not sharply distinguished in local usage. However, medical graduates of Ayurveda are now called doctors.

4 The Unani tradition of medicine came to Nepal through Islam and its traditional practitioners are usually referred to as *hakims*. Medical graduates of the Unani are also now called doctors.
5 The mechanistic paradigm describes the notion of the body as a machine, disease as the consequence of the breakdown of the machine, and the doctor's task as a repairer of the machine.

References

Baer, Hans A. et al. 1997. *Medical Anthropology and the World System*. Westport: Bergin and Gravey.

Barth, Fredrik. 1990. "The Guru and the Conjurer: Transactions in Knowledge and the Shaping of Culture in South-East Asia and Melanesia." *Man* 25: 640–653.

Barth, Fredrik. 1993. *Balinese Worlds*. Chicago: The University of Chicago Press.

Blustain, Harvey S. 1976. "Levels of Medicine in a Center Nepali Village." *Contributions to Nepalese Studies*. Special issue, 3. Center for Nepal and Asian Studies, Tribhuvan University, Kathmandu, Nepal.

Bourdieu, Pierre. 1977. *Outline of a Theory of Practice*. Cambridge: Cambridge University Press.

Christakis, Nicholas A. et al. 1994. "Illness Behaviour and Health Transition in the Developing World." In Lincoln C. Chen, ed., *Health and Social Change in International Perspective*. Harvard Series on Population and International Health. Cambridge, MA: Harvard University Press.

Devkota, Padam Lal. 1984. "Illness Interpretation and Modes of Treatment in Kirtipur." *Contributions to Nepalese Studies* 11(2): 11–20.

Dietrich, Angela. 1998. *Tantric Healing in Kathmandu Valley: A Comparative Study of Hindu and Buddhist Spiritual Healing Traditions in Urban Nepalese Society*. New Delhi: Book Faith India.

Dixit, Hemang. 1999. *The Quest for Health*. Kathmandu: Educational Enterprise (P) Ltd.

Durkin-Longley, Maureen. 1984. "Multiple Therapeutic Uses in Urban Nepal." *Social Science and Medicine* 19(8): 867–872.

Durkin-Longley, Maureen. 1988. "Ayurvedic Treatment for Jaundice in Nepal." *Social Science and Medicine* 27(5): 491–495.

Elias, Norbert. 1991. "On Human Beings and Their Emotions: A Process-Sociological Essay." In Mike Featherstone et al., eds., *The Body: Social Process and Cultural Theory*. London: Sage Publications.

Foster, George M. 1994. *Hippocrates' Latin American Legacy: Humoral Medicine in the New World*. New York: Gordon and Breach Science Publishers.

Foster, George M. and Barbara Anderson. 1978. *Medical Anthropology*. New York: John Wiley and Sons, Inc.

Geertz, Clifford. 1973. *The Interpretation of Culture*. New York: Basic Books.

Gellner, David N. 1994. "Priest, Healers, Mediums and Witches: The Context of Possession in Kathmandu Valley, Nepal." *Journal of Royal Anthropological Institute* 29(1): 27–48.

Goffman, Erving. 1959. *The Presentation of Self in Everyday Life*. New York: Doubleday Anchor Books.

Good, Byron J. 1994. *Medicine, Rationality and Experience: An Anthropological Perspective*. Cambridge: Cambridge University Press.

Helman, Cecil G. 1996. *Culture, Health and Illness: An Introduction for Health Professionals* (3rd Edition). Oxford: Butterworth-Heinemann.

Hitchock, John T. and Rex Jones, eds. 1976. *Spirit Possession in the Nepal Himalayas*. New Delhi: Vikas Publishing House.

Justice, Judith. 1986. *Policies, Plans, and People: Culture and Health Development in Nepal*. Berkeley: University of California Press.

Kleinman, Arthur. 1978. "Concepts and Model for the Comparison of Medical Systems as Cultural Systems." *Social Science and Medicine* 12: 85–93.

Kleinman, Arthur. 1980. *Patients and Healers in the Context of Culture*. Berkeley: University of California Press.

Kristvik, Ellen. 1999. *Drums and Syringes*. Bibliotheca Himalayica Series III, Vol. 7. Kathmandu: EMR.

Leslie, Charles, ed. 1976. *Asian Medical System: A Comparative Study*. Berkeley: University of California Press.

Leslie, Charles. 1978. "Pluralism and Integration in the Chinese Medical System." In A. Kleinman et al., eds., *Culture and Healing in Asian Societies*. Cambridge, MA: Schenkman Publishing Company.

Leslie, Charles. 1980. "Medical Pluralism in World Perspective." *Social Science and Medicine* 14B(4): 191–195.

Levitt, Marta. 1988. *From Sickle to Scissors: Birth, Traditional Birth Attendants and Perinatal Health Development in Rural Nepal*. Unpublished Ph. D. Thesis, University of Hawaii.

Lieban, Richard W. 1977. "The Field of Medical Anthropology." In David Landy, ed., *Culture, Disease and Healing: Studies in Medical Anthropology*. New York: Macmillan Publishing Co., Inc.

Macfarlane, Alan. 1994. "Fatalism and Development in Nepal." In Michael Hutt, ed., *Nepal in the Nineties – Versions of the Past, Visions of the Future*, pp. 106–127. Delhi: Oxford University Press.

Miller, Casper J. 1979. *Faith Healers in the Himalayas*. Kathmandu: Centre for Nepal and Asian Studies.

Ministry of Health. 2016. *Basic Information of Department of Ayurveda*. Kathmandu: Ministry of Health.

Minocha, Aneeta. 1980. "Medical Pluralism and Health Services in India." *Social Science and Medicine* 14B: 217–223.

NESAC. 1998. *Nepal Human Development Report 1998*. Kathmandu: Nepal South Asia Center.

Okada, Ferdinand. 1976. "Notes on Two Shamans-Curers in Kathmandu." *Contributions to Nepalese Studies*. Center for Nepal and Asian Studies, Tribhuvan University, Kathmandu, Nepal. Special issue, 3: 107–112.

Pelto, Pertii and Gretel Pelto. 1996. "Research Design in Medical Anthropology." In Sargent Carolyn F. and Thomas M. Johnson, eds., *Medical Anthropology: Contemporary Theory and Methods*. Praeger Publishers.

Pigg, Stacy Leigh. 1989. "Here, There and Every Where: Place and Person in Nepalese Explanations of Illness." *Himalayan Research Bulletin* 9(2): 16–23.

Pigg, Stacy Leigh. 1995. "Acronyms and Effacement: Traditional Medical Practitioners (TMP) in Internal Health Development." *Social Science and Medicine* 41(1): 47–68.

Shrestha, R. M. and M. Lediard. 1980. *Faith Healers: A Force for Change.* Kathmandu: UNFPA and UNICEF.

Stone, Linda. 1976. "Concept of Illness and Curing in a Central Nepal Village." *Contributions to Nepalese Studies.* Special issue, 3: 55–80. Center for Nepal and Asian Studies, Tribhuvan University, Kathmandu, Nepal.

Streefland, Pieter. 1985. "The Frontier of Modern Western Medicine in Nepal." *Social Science and Medicine* 20(11): 1151–1159.

Subedi, Janardan. 1988. *Factors Affecting the Use of Medicine in a Pluralistic Health Care System: The Case of Nepal.* Unpublished Ph. D. Thesis, University of Akron.

Subedi, Janardan. 1989. "Modern Health Services and Health Care Behavior: A Survey in Kathmandu, Nepal." *Journal of Health and Social Behavior* 30: 412–420.

Subedi, Madhusudan Sharma. 2001a. "Development and Underdevelopment of Modern Health Services in Nepal." *Deva Vani* 4: 217–224.

Subedi, Madhusudan Sharma. 2001b. *Medical Anthropology of Nepal.* Kathmandu: Udaya Books.

Wake, C. J. 1976. "Health Services and Some Cultural Factors in Urban Nepal." *Contributions to Nepalese Studies.* Special issue, 3: 113–125. Center for Nepal and Asian Studies, Tribhuvan University, Kathmandu, Nepal.

3 Illness causation and interpretation in a Newari town[1]

The objective of this chapter is to explore people's complex understanding of illness causation and interpretation. I argue that healing traditions are embedded with cosmos-genetic worldviews as parts of wider concepts about the origin of bodily afflictions in general. They are based on beliefs about the structure and functions of the body, and the ways in which it can function and malfunction. Even if based on biomedically incorrect premises, these explanations or models frequently have an integral logic and consistency which often helps the ill person to make sense of what has happened and why (Kleinman 1980; Helman 2002; Subedi 2001).

My argument is that people's ideas by which they explain and handle everyday life, partly are the same that they use to explain illness. By doing this, in my view, we will be able to better understand how people describe health and ill health. For example, what are the locally defined illnesses? What are thought to be the causes and the degree of severity and symptoms? What treatments are sought, and from whom? We will also be able to understand their explanation for their state of health, what they identify as important about themselves or their physical or social environment, and what, if anything, they believe can or should be done to protect or enhance their health.

Young (1983) has rightly pointed out that medical beliefs are the sets of premises and ideas that enable people to organize perceptions and experiences of their medical events and to organize their interventions for affecting and controlling these events. They are ways of defining problems and generating solutions to these problems. Following the arguments of Kleinman (1980); Helman (2002); Pigg (1989); and Subedi (2001), I argue that people's explanations for their illnesses show the complicated relationships that shape people's lives. Furthermore, by gaining an insider's perspective on culture, one can understand the notion of embodied personhood and its effect on the activities of sick people and their families, and the relationship between cultural beliefs, practices and health, ill health, and the sentient human body.

Methods and materials

This research was done in Kirtipur, called *Kipu* by the local Newars. Kirtipur is one of the oldest settlements in Nepal, located at the top of a hill in the Kathmandu Valley. The study area is inhabited by the Newars, living in a comparatively compact settlement characterized by the traditional social hierarchy according to which the Pradhans and Amatyas live in the central Layaku palace complex, followed by Shrestha and other middle-ranked caste groups. Maharjans, Manandhars, and Tandukaars and lower hierarchies are living on the outskirts. History says that the ancient city Kirtipur was founded by Shiva Deva between AD 1099 and AD 1126, and, during the reign of the Malla Kingdom in the 15th century, the city was further developed (Subedi 2001).

The research was designed to explore laypersons' understanding of the relationship between various types of ill health and symptoms and their perceptions of illness categories in relation to actual help-seeking behavior involving those illnesses.

The ethnographic work was done in July–December 1999, and in March 2010. The basic method of data collection was formal and informal discussions with elderly Newari males and females. During the discussions with elderly people, I was assisted by one Newari youth who could speak both Newari and Nepali. Some youths were included in the study to explore the variations in perceptions between the young and the old generations. Discussions with the elderly and the youths were done separately. A total of ten discussions were done during the visit in March 2010, six with elderly people and four with youths. The number of participants in the groups with elderly people ranged from three to six, and with youths from five to eight.

The aim for the research was to see things 'from the native point of view' or how local people feel and think in a changing context. It was an attempt to discover the meaning of what people chose to tell in the particular context of Kirtipur with all its distinct natural, social, and cultural properties. The interviews were not done in order to test a particular theoretical proposition. I did not know what I would find. During the interview, I attempted to be as neutral as possible, to allow people to speak without interruptions, and to remain open to unanticipated avenues related to their health, illness, and causes of ill health. Furthermore, I also wanted to explore whether the Newars in Kirtipur shared a 'bag of something called culture' (Haaland 2002) different from the cultural bags shared by other ethnic groups. If the ideas among the same ethnic group vary over time and generations, the members of a particular group thus entertain different ideas among themselves that are learned through social interaction. The broader social, cultural, political, and economic conditions contextualize the understanding and experiences of health and illness. This aspect of culture highlights its dynamic, changing quality and gives weight to the forces of change and interaction (Trostle 2005). From this perspective, culture is constantly being transformed.

Findings and discussions

The understanding of bodily affliction in Kirtipur, as in any other community, goes far beyond exploring the ambiguous causes and their appropriate remedies (Foster and Anderson 1978; Stone 1976; Devkota 1984; Pigg 1995; Helman 2002). The understanding of people's life and world, their conceptions of a healthy person and illness causality stems from a distinctive conceptual organization of social interaction (Okada 1976). People always present logical, rational explanations for illnesses (causes and consequences), and curing techniques are organized accordingly within the local cultural perspective and social organization (Devkota 1984; Nepali 1965) but may also be influenced by other cultures.

People's life and the world

Almost all elderly males and females in Kirtipur mentioned that there is a vital force, *shakti*, a power or energy for balancing the whole universe. God is the source of power. In order to appease the god, people have to perform rituals and make sacrifices. They mentioned that the various rituals such as birth initiation, marriage, and death are activities that link the visible and invisible world. The visible world is easy to look at, hear, or feel. The invisible world, according to them, was a complex one. Their understanding was that whatever happened to the individual in life was strongly linked to the invisible world. On the other hand, the youths, although not highlighting the power of the invisible world, could not deny it either. They did, however, emphasize the physical world more.

Conceptions of a healthy person

Almost all informants mentioned that they considered their children to be healthy if they are well and not ill. Eating well as usual, smiling when looking at other faces, sleeping well, and defecating and urinating well were the frequently cited features of a healthy child. Some respondents mentioned the proper growth of a child as one of the most important indicators of being healthy. Inability to eat and sleep, coughing and having a fever, crying, loss of weight all were the features of an unhealthy child. Both the elderly and the youths had a similar understanding of the concept of a healthy and unhealthy child. Digestion capacity of various types of food was perceived as one of the major indicators of a healthy person, followed by memory capacity, positive attitude towards others, eating and sleeping well, and gaining height and weight. Ill health is usually linked as part of a much wider set of options for explaining 'bad luck', 'misfortune', and 'carelessness'. The elderly people highlighted misfortune and bad luck, while the youths were more concerned with carelessness, poverty, social discrimination, and exclusion.

The concept of 'strong health' and 'weak health' was also linked with the health of the mother. "A weak mother cannot give a healthy baby," was a frequently mentioned response. Likewise, the mother's carelessness during pregnancy was also linked to a weak child. The youths also highlighted the importance of prenatal care and the necessity to visit biomedical practitioners. The elderly, on the other hand, focused on worshiping gods and goddesses, preferring specific food, and to continue the household work to deliver a healthy child. Some respondents expressed the belief that the strengths and weaknesses of a baby depended on the nature and function of the husband's as well as the wife's blood. An occasional weakness, headache, pain in the stomach, back, or in other parts of the body were taken as normal problems. They were linked to occupational work and seen as temporary problems. Taking a rest for a few hours was a commonly cited response to return back to the normal condition.

Illness causation

The participants were asked to describe illnesses they had experienced during their lifetime and to consider the causes of these illnesses. In general, etiology or causation of ill health was interpreted in terms of one of the four different worlds: within the individual, in the natural world, in the social world, and in the supernatural world. In many cases, people perceived the illness as the combination of two or more causes, or as the interaction between these various worlds (Helman 2002).

Individual carelessness was a frequently cited cause for ill health. People perceived the origin of ill health as malfunctions within the body and that these were linked to changes in the diet or behavior. Thus, the responsibility for illnesses fell mainly, though not completely, on the patients themselves. Ill health was increasingly seen as caused by the people 'not taking care' of one's diet, clothing, hygiene, sexual behavior, smoking habits, and physical exercise. Illness was, therefore, often perceived as evidence of such carelessness, and the sufferer felt guilty for causing it. According to Helman (2002), such lay explanations are also common in the western world. In order to prevent and cure these health problems, people suggested a change in their food habits and other behaviors such as personal hygiene, keeping the house clean, and washing clothes regularly. The young and educated respondents mentioned that obesity, sexually transmitted diseases, drug dependency, diabetic, and heart-related diseases resulted from incorrect behavior or individual carelessness. Doing something abnormal such as walking without an umbrella during rain or hot weather, walking without slippers during the summer and winter, eating salty and heavy food in the evening, doing heavy work during menstruation and immediately after delivery, drinking too much alcohol and chain-smoking, having an unsafe sexual relationship, and using drugs were some of the frequently cited individual behaviors causing ill health. Some participants also mentioned personal vulnerability, arguing that different people have different types of physical vulnerability. "Some people are physically stronger and more resistant to illness than others," they said. Some of the respondents said: "Many children suffer from dental problems due to their food habits. They do not prefer traditional food like roasted maize, bread, green vegetables and pulses but prefer a variety of junk food, sweets and candies."

Most of the study's participants linked nature and environment with illness. The natural world thought to cause ill health included aspects of the natural environment, both living and inanimate. Ill health could be caused by climatic conditions such as extreme cold, heat, wind, rain, water pollution, air pollution, or by parasitic infection and accidental injuries.

Blaming other people for one's ill health is common in many societies where interpersonal conflicts are frequent (Helman 2002). In Kirtipur, the most frequent reasons for this type were *bokshi* and *aankha* (evil eyes). The *bokshis* in Nepal are thought to be the chief causes of any kind of affliction. The complex belief associated with the *bokshi* is unambiguously feminine and considered as humans, unlike the other manifestations of the supernatural sphere. Elderly people mentioned that it is religiously wrong to discuss *bokshis* at all, and that in doing so, they attract their malign attention. On the other hand, youths were not aware of this issue. They simply said that they had heard the words *bokshi* and *aankha*.

Some informants said that *bokshis* go near the cremation ground and worship the goddess without clothing, thus obtaining power. They can turn into animals at will. In this sense *bokshis*, of course, are human, but symbolically they are like an extension of violent and dangerous aspects of the goddess in the human world. These females are said to become devotees of goddesses so that they can send her to attack others with illness or barrenness. Anyone who harms others by magical means is considered a *bokshi* who act on an item of clothing or hair of the victim. But a *bokshi* may also harm simply by looking at people, particularly at the food they eat. Some elderly female respondents said that anyone can do this, while others said it only happens if the onlooker desires to harm. Consensus regarding the *bokshi* activities could not be found even among the elderly women. The context in which *bokshis* are encountered is the actual suspicion and naming of known people. In practice it is women, especially old women, and among them especially widows, who are suspected of being *bokshis*. There are some marked similarities with the description of *bokshis* in other countries (Landy 1977), and also among other groups in Nepal (Stone 1976; Gellner 1994; Kristvik 1999).

The problem of controlling a *bokshi* is left to the *Janne Manchhe*, *Jharphuke Vaidya*, *Dhami*, *Jhankri*, and *Gubhaju* who are supposed to be well versed in counteracting her evil doings. They employ many ways to punish her. People believe that *Jharphuke Vaidya*, *Janne Manchhe*, *Dhami*, *Jhankri*, or *Gubhaju* catch her through the afflicted person, to reveal her identity, and to state the reason for evil doings. As a mild course, a healer merely asks her to free the man or woman and promises that she never again will possess him/her. In this case they would not reveal her identity. In some cases, the *Janne Manchhe* takes stern measures, such as branding the afflicted person's body with spots with a red-hot iron. This burn is supposed to be transferred to the body of the *bokshi* and people believed that the *bokshi* in question would be found with an identical burn. Sometimes dried chilly is burnt and it is believed that its smoke would suffocate the *bokshi* who would come running to the place. In some cases, it was believed that the *Janne Manchhe*, by uttering incantations, causes his client to vomit blood, resulting in actual blood being vomited by the *bokshi* at her place. However, I could not confirm these cases in Kirtipur.

There are different ways of punishing *bokshis*. News about *bokshi* frequently appears in the newspapers as well as in other social media. There are, in my view, thousands of such cases in Nepal, which

go unnoticed, unreported, or under-reported. Depending on the availability and belief of the different ethnic groups in Nepal, healers like
Dhami, Jhankri, Gubhaju, Janne Manchhe, Jharphuke, Ma, and many
others use their own method to punish the *bokshis* and to drive the
spirit of the *bokshi* away. If a child, another person, or cattle die, a
woman is targeted as a *bokshi* who is perceived as having caused these
deaths. She is beaten, humiliated, and forced to feed on human feces.
If she survives at all, unable to bear the insult, she hardly ventures out
of her house (Subedi 2001). Several media have frequently reported
that women in different districts have been fed human excreta on the
charge of being a *bokshi*.

Elderly people in Kirtipur believed that there was a close a connection between *Janne Manchhe* and *bokshis*. It is often said that the
knowledge which the *Janne Manchhe* must have is the same, only
stronger than that of the *bokshis*. *Janne Manchhe* knows how to cause
harm, and how to undo it. Many healers are believed to have mas-
tered the *bokshi* mantra in order to combat evil powers. Likewise,
bokshis are thought to have healing capabilities. The basic knowledge
is the same whether it is *subidhya* (good knowledge) or *kubidhya* (bad
knowledge); the healing depends on how it is used. Some people said
that a female *Janne Manchhe* is the same as *bokshi*. There seemed to
be an agreement that *Janne Manchhe* and *bokshi* hold the same kind
of power, but the *Janne Manchhe* was said to have one mantra more
than the *bokshi*, which gave them the upper hand.

The youths in Kirtipur had different attitudes towards *bokshis* and
supernatural powers. They gave different responses to the idea of *Dhami,
Jhankri,* or *Janne Manchhe*. Traditionally, *Dhami,* and *Jhankri* are supposed to be psychic healers and are hence seen with both respect and
fear in rural parts of the country (Allen 1976; Peters 1979; Maskarinec 1995; Miller 1997).

As far as healing goes, the *Jhankris* do enjoy some degree of respect
mainly due to ignorance among people. The youths said that pointing
out *bokshis* and persecuting them at times even to the point of killing
them or making them commit suicide simply could not be allowed.
The *Dhami, Jhankri,* or *Janne Manchhe*, whoever it was, should be
punished. According to the young people, this was one of the ways
to measure the country's backwardness. Some educated young persons and human right activists mentioned that superstition reflects the
predominance of illiteracy and ignorance among people. The *Dhami,
Jhankri,* or any types of healer who point out a woman as *bokshi* were
garlanded with money. My informants further argued that the superstitious belief of feeding human excreta to women on the charge of

being a *bokshi* still continued because the culturally constructed ideas were deeply rooted in the minds of the Nepali people.

Belief in the spiritual world was very strong among the Newars as well as among other inhabitants of the valley or in the country as a whole (Nepali 1965; Hitchcock and Jones 1976; Stone 1976; Blustain 1976; Devkota 1984; Pigg 1995; Gellner 1994). Kathmandu is the city of gods and goddesses and the haunting place of spirits and ghosts. Almost all the elderly, discussion participants in Kirtipur believed that these *bhut, pret, khya*, and other hungry ghosts could bring disease and death to those who neglect them, blight to crops, fires to houses, barrenness to wives, and disease and drought to the village. The elderly people classified the god and goddess, demon, *bhut* (ghost), *pret, masan*, and *bayu* as supernatural beings. The notion of the *shakti* (power) was the defining characteristic of supernatural beings. The basic characteristic of any god, demon or ghost was the power that he/she controls and represents, the fact that he/she was, in essence, power.

Given the premise that "supernatural beings are powerful beings," I will describe the roles underlying the ascription of power, the behavior of power-filled beings, and thereby ritual behavior, by examining the way in which power was used, explained and dealt with by the people. This includes two related questions: How did local people perceive the ways in which these powers were distributed among their deities? How did powerful beings function in controlling the relevant aspect of life?

The noun in Nepali that comes close to including all possible powerful beings is *devi, devata*, which is defined to include gods and goddesses. The common characteristic of all Kirtipur deities is *shakti* (power). The Nepali term closest in meaning to *shakti* is *bal*, but *bal* implies a physical strength in contrast to *shakti*, which implies a spiritual power, although that spiritual power can be manifested physically. Thus a person is said to have *bal* but not necessarily *shakti*, and the gods have *shakti* but not necessarily *bal*. Temples and shrines are supposed to be *shakti griha* (power stations) but only spiritual powerhouses. Each item of the universe has its share of *shakti* (power). Wadley (1975: 55) noted: "Every genus of living beings shares from the moment of its generation its defining qualities (*guna*), powers (*shakti*), and actions (*karma*)." Thus every being of the universe embodies its share of power, but some beings have more power than others (Dietrich 1998). Those beings with more *shakti* are the powerful beings (supernatural beings), beings with less *shakti* are not so powerful. Moreover, because every being in the universe by definition embodies some power, everything in the universe is potentially a powerful being.

However, all gods and goddesses and other supernatural beings are not equally powerful.

An examination of a few Kirtipur deities should clarify this point. Bagh Bhairav, Indriyani, Uma-Maheshwar, Ganesh, Shiva, Laxmi, and Saraswati are at any time and in any place powerful. There are shrines and statues for all these deities and people offer regular *puja* (worship) for them on auspicious days. These deities do not inflict illness on an individual without reasons. They are the protective forces for places and people. If an individual offends them, he/she suffers from illness. Under such circumstances, he/she prays to these deities to be saved from their designs. They may promise the *puja* (worship) to the affiliated deity at a later date, which must be fulfilled. These deities may withhold their protection for an individual being attacked by evil forces. Thus villagers offer regular offerings or worship. The Bagh Bhairav Temple is dedicated to the Bhairav god in the form of a tiger. This god is regarded as the guardian of Kirtipur and the locals call it *Ajudeu*, a grandfather god. Likewise, a boy and a girl, as groom and bride, are recognized during the marriage ceremonies as god and goddess. In Kirtipur, they are considered Ram and Sita – so much so that their elders touch their feet.

People in general believed that all the gods and goddesses affected their life, although their shrines were located outside their villages. Harati ma, a goddess of smallpox and measles, whose shrine is at Swyambhu in Kathmandu, is worshiped regularly. Even though smallpox in Nepal has been eradicated, this practice is continuing even today. Similarly, Khayatama Deo (the protector of children) of Bhat-Bhateni is also worshiped in return for protection. The Unmateshwar Bhairav of Gyaneshwar, Sankkata Deo of Tebahal, Bijeshwari of Shobha Bhagati, Matshe Narayan of Machhe Gaon, and several other gods and goddess are also worshiped so that they can continue to protect people. Machhendranath is considered as the provider of rain and grain to the Kathmandu Valley. Likewise, one can see a round plate of stone on the doorstep of most Newari houses, it being regarded as a symbol of Kumar, the son of Shiva and Parbati. This worship is done before any other daily household worship, and is common only among the Newaris.

Almost all the elderly discussion participants mentioned that the gods, ghosts, and demons have various kinds of powers that might control human conditions. Similarly, a bride and groom are power-filled because they represent fertility and prosperity, the future growth of the family. A snake is powerful because it can kill. All that exists in the universe contains some power and can be part of a Hindu pantheon. Thus, when discussing the Newari cultural conceptions, we must recognize that there is no native conception of a bounded regional domain on the spiritual. People believed that gods and goddesses are superior to human beings and thus must be worshiped. In return, they bestow benefits on human beings.

Worship of *nagas* (serpent gods) was common among the Newaris. The traditional story is that when Manjushree drained the lake, the then Kathmandu, most *nagas* left the abode except for one *Karkotaka naga* who today is believed to dwell in *Tau Daha*, a lake in the southern outskirts of the valley. It was because of *Karkotaka naga* that the valley retained the water and did not turn completely dry (Nepali 1965; Gurung 2000). In the events of drought, Newaris in Kirtipur go to *Tau Daha* and worship *Karkotaka*. When one gets rashes on the body, one needs to worship the *nagas*. The elderly people believed that the *nagas* ensured peace, bestowed riches, and protected the house. The youths were not aware of this type of explanation of *nagas* and their role for peace and protection.

The ghost-like creatures, associated with the spirits of the dead, are often called *pret* or *bhut-pret* (from the Sanskrit term *preta*, locally pronounced *pret*). *Pret* refers to the particular spiritual principle or entity that represents the continuation of a person after death, undergoing various transformations. For the first 12 days after death the spirit is perceived to be in a *pret* form. *Pret* is variously perceived as being an ancestor spirit or *pitr*, being safely on its way to some place of judgment, or in a state of reincarnation. The corpse is also referred to as *pret*. There are various mishaps that can prevent the proper passage through and beyond the *pret* stage, and the *pret* then will become a troublesome earth-bound ghost. A person who is not ready to die or do not want to may become a permanent *pret*. A common notion among the elderly was that "Someone who dies in such a way that the proper ritual cannot be done – such as an accident away from the home or whose death is considered unnatural – can also become such a *pret*."

The presence of these ghosts is often harmlessly manifested in such events as a window or door moving by itself or a chair shifting position. They usually stay around their former homes, and will not harm family members if as many as possible of the proper post-death rituals have been performed. Similarly, the ghosts and spirits cluster at crossroads, inhabit the woods and fields outside the city, lurk in the dark, and are driven away by bright lights. Sometimes they may invade a home but usually in outside shadowy areas. An encounter with them is usually a matter of some accidents or inadvertent mistake. There are, however, more malevolent varieties that may enter a person and consume him/her from the inside, causing him/her to lose weight and become ill, requiring the service of special exorcists of spirits.

There are still other beings that for some people are kinds of *bhuts*, for others, kinds of *prets*, and, for still others, neither *pret* nor *bhut*, but independent beings. Among these is the *Khya*, which exists in two forms, white and black. The white is benign and guards the house from other spirits. It sometimes may snuggle up to a person, and produce a tickling feeling. The black ones may produce frightening nightmares. They may press on people's chest during sleep, making it difficult to breathe or to move. For some people *Khyas* are independent spirits, but not *bhuts*, for others they are a kind of *bhut*, and for still others they arise from a body that has not been thoroughly cremated so that some flesh remains.

Similarly, the stone and the crossing roads, and the divinity thought to be located there are called *chhwasa*. The *chhwasa* is sometimes considered as a divinity in itself, at other times among the more erudite as the seat of the tantric goddesses, Matangi. Some old respondents mentioned that *chhwasa* is related to the death spirit of the family, the grandfather and the grandmother (*aju-aji*). The belief is that *aju-aji* attacks human beings only when their hunger is not appeased. When one suspects their attack, the hunger must be satisfied, offering them a small share. It is believed that small children are most vulnerable, but *aju-aji* can attack adults too. The Kirtipur informants said that sudden stomach pain, headache, bleeding through the mouth, and diarrhea were key signs and symptoms of an attack by *aju-aji*.

The *chhwasa* is one of the places where polluting materials are deposited so that they no longer will be dangerous or problematic. The clothes worn by a person at the time of or just before death are gathered and thrown to the *chhwasa*. Certain remains of formal feasts are discarded there. The *chhwasa* lies at a crossroad and is thought to be a gathering place for potentially harmful spirits. It is also the place where people discard cloths soiled by menstruation, the umbilical cords of newborn infants, clothes of the dead, and food as offering to potentially harmful spirits. The *chhwasa* not only can observe the polluted materials placed on it and the materials that would be strongly contaminating if placed in any ordinary space within the city, but is also said to protect the area around it (Devkota 1984). However, my observations showed that the practice of throwing polluted materials at the *chhwasa* has decreased compared to past. This may be due to the practice of collecting garbage by the Kirtipur Municipality. The main *chhwasa* was said to protect the entire village. This combination of power to absorb polluting materials and to protect is a general characteristic of a class of dangerous deities, the *chhwasa* being one of them.

Mental health and symbolic healing

Loss of memory, repetitive activities, aggressiveness, misbehaving with family members and friends, dramatic changes in eating and sleeping habits, poor grades despite hard work and strong efforts, damaging property are all seen as problems related to *dimag* (mental). When such things happen, the patient is surrounded by family and friends. The mental illnesses are explained in terms of possession by *bhut*, *pret*, *pisach*, *bayu*, *bokshi*, and gods. This is also linked to a person's bad *karma*, *bhagya*, and *mohini*. Similar findings are stated in Jirels of Jiri (Tausig et al. 2000).

The people who participated in the discussions in Kirtipur had a negative attitude towards mentally suffering persons, often stigmatizing them. The suffering individual was taken to the *Dhami*, *Jhankri*, and *Janne Manchhe*, and to various temples for worshiping the gods and goddesses. Many elderly people held the view that such problems were hereditary. Those people being aware of mental illness thought that it was different from other types of health problems such as accidents and fractures, a fever, or vomiting, all of which could be cured. They believed that mental illness might occur repeatedly. The youths mentioned that such problems often are cured by visiting a psychiatrist, worshiping the gods and goddesses, and visiting the local healers.

Health seeking behavior

The participants in the discussions in Kirtipur shared their illness experiences from their childhood and consistently and repeatedly mentioned that, in the past, people used to practice home-based self-medication, to use various types of herbs, and changing their diet. Visiting the doctor was very uncommon unless the symptoms of illness were very serious or unless someone was almost dead. Elderly discussion participants were keen to tell the interviewer that they were very critical of the contemporary view of treatment among the younger generations: "When anyone is not feeling well with a minor wound, ache or pain, they immediately visit the doctor." Elderly people seemed to be particularly critical of their children and grandchildren's amount of, as well as the causes for, contacting allopathic medical practitioners. They said that allopathic medicine is effective sometimes, but that it can become habitual for a person. Their opinion was that once a person starts to take allopathic medicine, herbal, or other types of indigenous medicine do not work. They also thought that the continuous use of allopathic medicine for one disease and then for another disease made a person weak, and possibly more prone to catch another type of disease.

On the other hand, the youths were not that much critical of allopathic medicine. When comparing the patterns of help seeking in Kirtipur in 1999 and 2010, I found some differences. In 1999, there were few medical shops in Kirtipur. In 2010, there was a hospital, about a dozen multi-purpose clinics, and many medical shops in the expanded town, Naya Bazar, and its surrounding areas. Over-the-counter medicine had become very common, followed by the practice of consulting the paramedics and the general practitioners. There were about half a dozen dental clinics, and an Ayurvedic Hospital about 20 minutes walking distance from the old town of Kirtipur.

Elderly people said that they sought specific healers based on the nature of their illness symptoms. They did not always blame the victims themselves, and sometimes people were unable to find any reason for blaming another person for ill health. For example, Newaris in Kirtipur considered a twitch of a muscle (*sarko*) to be caused by disequilibrium inside the human body. To cure the illness, they consulted a *Janne Manchhe* who knew the correct spell (*sarko mantra*). On the other hand, the young people said that they would visit the medical shop or allopathic healer for the treatment of such problems. They also mentioned that they would visit the *Janne Manchhe* and at the same time continue with the medicine that had been bought in a medical shop.

There was a similar situation regarding another illness called *Janaikai* in Kirtipur. In the classical Newari language, the term *janai* means a sacred cord worn by the twice-born castes in Nepal and *kai* means infected wounds (*khatira-patira*) on the skin (Devkota 1984). The *janaikai* appears as boils on the body in a circular form like a sacred cord. The stomach, the waist, and the chest are the bodily parts where *janaikai* usually appears. The part where the boils appear first is called *chyo* (head) and where it appears last is known as *nyaphyo* (tail). Local people believed that when the boils complete a circle, the person might die. Therefore, when it appeared, the person immediately must consult a painter or *chitrakar*. This person draws two figures of the lion (one at the head and another at the tail of the infected area) with an ordinary ink pen. In both figures, the open mouth of the lion faces the boils. People believed that these two figures of the lion would swallow the boils and within a few days the disease would disappear. However, the youths mentioned that people's perception that ill health is caused by their own behavior depended on a number of socio-economic factors over which the individual had no control.

In general, elderly people started home-based self-medication to recover as early as possible. Health can be seen as a state of equilibrium in which the balance is maintained according to the individual's age and condition in the natural and social environment. Some youths said that an illness is triggered by an upset in a balance between, for instance, hot and cold, and that excessive heat or cold had entered the body. Treatment logically attempts to restore the balance through hot and cold food, and the treatment aims at neutralizing either excessive heat or cold from the body.

The elderly also believed that diseases are caused by an imbalance of certain elements within the body, for instance, between air and water. A person who has a balanced bodily constitution between hot and cold is less liable to ailment and illness. In order to restore the balance between cold and hot, they must eat food or take traditional medicine that has the opposite characteristic, for instance, eating hot food during the cold season and vice versa. The elderly people believed that diarrhea is related to the food consumed by the lactating mother, and that it is transmitted to the baby through the mother's milk when she eats certain cold foods that should be avoided during lactation. The youths, however, did not have such views.

Expansion of biomedicine in Kirtipur

Allopathic medicine has been practiced in Nepal from the middle of the 18th century. According to Dixit (1995), the first reference to allopathic practitioners in this country occurs in an account of the siege of Kirtipur by King Prithvi Narayan Shah in 1766–1767. It was Swarup Ratna, the King's brother, who had been cured of a wound by one Michael Angelo, a Capuchin monk.

Prithvi Bir Hospital, the first allopathic public hospital in Nepal was built in 1890 in Kathmandu, at the northwestern corner of Ranipokhari. The total number of beds was only 30. Currently, many private hospitals and medical colleges are established in almost all towns in Nepal. The health sector has been one of the most successful businesses in the private sector. Over-the-counter medicine and non-doctor prescriptions have been very common also in Kirtipur. My study registered that prescriptions and the use of antibiotics were rampant, and that patients took half of the doses of medicine as an attitude of wait and see. Visiting the medical shop of *afno manche* (kin group or relatives), followed by going to trustworthy persons and hospitals were more common.

For the last 25 years I have been observing Kirtipur as a student and researcher, and as a permanent resident. The allopathic health care system has been blooming rapidly in Kirtipur. Consulting the government doctors and private hospitals outside Kirtipur has become more common, and biomedicine has become significantly more popular for diagnosis and treatment. Health care has been commodified and commercialized, and the poor has to find cheaper services.

Conclusion

The perceptions of a healthy person and the processes of becoming ill consist of a combination of subjective experiences of physical or emotional changes, and the confirmation of these changes by other people. The study in Kirtipur showed that one easily can observe the different, although quite complex, conceptions of a healthy and unhealthy body, to understand illness causation, and interpret preventive as well as curative healing practices.

The understanding of illness etiology and health seeking behavior among the Newaris in Kirtipur was linked to several causes and health care practices acting together. This means that individual, natural, social, and supernatural causes were not mutually exclusive, but were usually linked together in a particular case. In any specific case of illness, people emphasized different causes when they attempted to explain its etiology. Moreover, explanations varied according to age and to the exposure of various medical traditions and practices, especially allopathic medicine.

This clearly shows that the members of particular groups reflect different health beliefs and practices among themselves. Belief and practices are not consistent essential features to understand bodily afflictions and their cure within certain ethnic groups. Cultural categories not only change through time, but they also can be manipulated differently by people interacting within a web of relationships that are embedded in a larger material and social context. Such knowledge is essential for developing more appropriate health policies, deepening our understanding of disease causation and treatment, and for creating more effective actions to enhance health and prevent disease.

Note

1 A version of this chapter originally appeared as 'Illness Causation and Interpretation in a Newar Town', *Dhaulagiri Journal of Sociology and Anthropology*, 5: 101–120, 2011. Used with permission.

References

Allen, Nicholas. 1976. "Shamanism among the Thulung Rai." In John T. Hitchcock and Rex L. Jones, eds., *Spirit Possession in the Nepal Himalaya*, pp. 124–140. New Delhi: Vikas Publishing Press.

Blustain, Harvey S. 1976. "Levels of Medicine in a Center Nepali Village." *Contributions to Nepalese Studies* 3: 83–105.

Devkota, Padam Lal. 1984. "Illness Interpretation and Modes of Treatment in Kirtipur." *Contributions to Nepalese Studies* 11(2): 11–20.

Dietrich, Angela. 1998. *Tantric Healing in Kathmandu Valley: A Comparative Study of Hindu and Buddhist Spiritual Healing Traditions in Urban Nepalese Society*. New Delhi: Book Faith India.

Dixit, Hemang. 1995. *The Quest for Health*. Kathmandu: Educational Enterprise (P) Ltd.

Foster, George and Barbara Anderson. 1978. *Medical Anthropology*. New York: John Wiley and Sons, Inc.

Gellner, David N. 1994. "Priest, Healers, Mediums and Witches: The Context of Possession in Kathmandu Valley, Nepal." *Journal of Royal Anthropological Institute* 29(1): 27–48.

Gurung, Poonam. 2000. *Bungmati: The Life World of Newar Community Explored through the Natural and Social Life of Water*. Unpublished Thesis, Faculty of Social Science, University of Bergen, Bergen, Norway.

Haaland, Gunnar. 2002. "Culture, Society and Nature: Reflection on Some Contribution from the Arun Valley." In Ram P. Chaudhary, Bhim P. Subedi, Ole R. Vetaas and Tor H. Aase, eds., *Vegetation and Society: Their Interaction in the Himalayas*, pp. 191–200. Kathmandu: Tribhuvan University and Bergen, Norway: University of Bergen.

Helman, Cecil G. 2002. *Culture, Health and Illness* (4th Edition). London: Arnold.

Hitchcock, John T. and Rex Jones, eds. 1976. *Spirit Possession in the Nepal Himalayas*. New Delhi: Vikas Publishing House.

Kleinman, Arthur. 1980. *Patients and Healers in the Contexts of Culture*. Berkeley: University of California Press.

Kristvik, Ellen. 1999. *Drums and Syringes*. Bibliotheca Himalayica Series III, Vol. 7. Kathmandu: EMR.

Landy, David, ed. 1977. "Traditional Curer under the Impact of Western Medicine." In *Culture, Disease and Healing: Studies in Medical Anthropology*. New York: Macmillan Publishing Co., Inc.

Maskarinec, Gregory G. 1995. *The Rulings of the Night: An Ethnography of Nepalese Shaman Oral Texts*. Kathmandu: Mandala Book Point.

Miller, Casper J. 1997. *Faith Healers in the Himalaya*. New Delhi: Book Faith India.

Nepali, Gopal Singh. 1965. *The Newars: An Ethno-Sociological Study of a Himalayan Community*. Bombay: United Asia Publication.

Okada, Ferdinand. 1976. "Notes on Two Shamans-Curers in Kathmandu." *Contributions to Nepalese Studies*. Special issue, 3: 107–112.

Peters, Larry G. 1979. "Shamanism and Medicine in Developing Nepal." *Contributions to Nepalese Studies* 6(2): 27–43.

Pigg, Stacy Leigh. 1989. "Here, There and Every Where: Place and Person in Nepalese Explanations of Illness." *Himalayan Research Bulletin* 9(2): 16–23.

Pigg, Stacy Leigh. 1995. "Acronyms and Effacement: Traditional Medical Practitioners (TMP) in Internal Health Development." *Social Science and Medicine* 41(1): 47–68.

Stone, Linda. 1976. "Concept of Illness and Curing in a Central Nepal Village." *Contributions to Nepalese Studies*. Special issue, 3: 55–80.

Subedi, Madhusudan. 2001. *Medical Anthropology of Nepal*. Kathmandu: Udaya Books.

Tausig, Mark et al. 2000. "Mental Illness in Jiri, Nepal." *Contributions to Nepalese Studies*. Special issue: 105–115.

Trostle, James A. 2005. *Epidemiology and Culture*. Cambridge Studies in Medical Anthropology. Cambridge: Cambridge University Press.

Wadley, Susan Snow. 1975. *Power in the Conceptual Structure of Karimpur Religion*. University of Chicago Studies in Anthropology. Chicago: Department of Anthropology, University of Chicago.

Young, Allan. 1983. "The Relevance of Traditional Medical Cultures to Modern Primary Health Care." *Social Science and Medicine* 17(16): 1205–1211.

4 Indigenous knowledge and health development in Nepal[1]

Two of the greatest barriers to the provision of primary health care in developing countries are the cost and shortage of trained staff (Gillam 1989). In Nepal, as elsewhere, patients choose from a wide range of options for dealing with illness: from self-treatment, to traditional and, finally, to allopathic medicine. Many patients seek care from several different systems simultaneously or at different stages during an illness period. These choices often represent highly rational responses to the constraints and opportunities people face. By selecting from several alternative sources of health care, people obtain therapies at an affordable cost (Subedi 2001).

People very well know many aspects of their surroundings and their daily lives. Over centuries, people have learned how to grow food and how to survive in difficult environments. They know about various types of food that are given for different illnesses (e.g. fever, cough and colds, diarrhea, skin infection, etc.), about beliefs regarding feeding the sick, classifications of plants that are poisonous and which can be used for medicine, how to cure diseases, and how to maintain their environment in a state of equilibrium (IIRR 1996).

This chapter reviews the literature about these issues, but does not purport to provide a comprehensive picture of indigenous health care in Nepal. The focus is on the importance of indigenous health care in Nepal, arguing for the government, particularly the Ministry of Health and Population (MoHP), to be interested in this subject by identifying the major policy issues that the government should seek to address.

Indigenous knowledge is the knowledge that people in a given community have developed over time, and continue to develop. It is based on experience, often tested over centuries, and adapted to local cultures and environments. It is not confined to specific castes or ethnic groups within particular areas nor even confined to rural people. Rather, any community possesses indigenous knowledge – rural and urban, settled and nomadic, original inhabitants, and migrants (IIRR 1996). Indigenous knowledge involves the process of experimentation, adoption, and development (Gill 1993). There are various concepts and terms related to indigenous knowledge; local knowledge, folk knowledge, rural people's knowledge, traditional knowledge, popular knowledge, non-western knowledge, emic knowledge, and ethno-science (Kamanta 2000). These terms are closely related, and it can be difficult to distinguish between them. In this chapter I have not differentiated between the words 'indigenous', 'local', or 'traditional', although not necessarily being the same.

Indigenous knowledge is a valuable resource for social development, including promoting good health, and under certain circumstances being equal or even superior to the know-how introduced by outsiders (IIRR 1996). Although more and more development professionals realize the potential of indigenous knowledge, it still remains a neglected resource. A key reason is the lack of guidelines for recording and applying indigenous knowledge. Without such guidelines, there is a danger that it will become just another empty buzzword of the sort that litters the history of development efforts (IIRR 1996). There is no single approach to recording indigenous knowledge, nor do I claim to have invented the methods described.

The attitudes and behaviors of the development practitioners, or the 'outsiders', are also important. Professionals must face the challenge of un-learning previous assumptions, which imply that the modern often must replace the traditional. Outsiders must be open and willing to learn from indigenous people. At the same time, local people, or the insiders, must learn to appreciate and value their indigenous knowledge. When people disregard their own knowledge, traditional wisdom, and practices are slowly lost. To make indigenous knowledge effective, all involved must recognize its usefulness and potential.

Understanding indigenous knowledge is fundamental to participatory development approaches. However, we need to go one step beyond just understanding indigenous knowledge. We must actively search for and identify indigenous knowledge that can be relevant for the planning, implementation, monitoring, and evaluation of specific projects. This means employing local healers, using traditional education methods, preserving and multiplying indigenous tree species, working with local organizations, and spreading messages through indigenous communication channels – to give only a few possibilities. At the same time, we must recognize that actively promoting selected indigenous technologies and practices does not necessarily make development participatory. For example, a project can introduce indigenous herbal medicine in a village without first consulting the local people. Villagers might, or might not, decide to use the herbal drugs, depending on the how the project as a whole is presented, whether it is culturally appropriate, and so on. Only if the active application of indigenous knowledge is part of a people-centered, truly participatory development effort, will it be possible to realize the potentials of indigenous knowledge in development processes. Indigenous knowledge draws on local resources, and people are less dependent on outside supplies that can be costly, scarce, and irregularly available. Thus, indigenous knowledge is very important for the poor who, having limited access to resources in their local community, should be encouraged to feel a sense of legitimacy regarding their knowledge and beliefs.

Indigenous healing traditions

The study of indigenous healing is important for sociologists and anthropologists as well as being the chief concern of clinicians who pursue cross-cultural research. They seek to elucidate universal as well as culturally particular features of the healing process, and they wish to compare indigenous healing with professional medical and psychiatric care (Kleinman and Sung 1979). The chief research questions are straightforward and have been known for quite some time. Is indigenous healing effective? If so, how? What role do cultural factors play in bringing about efficacy? How does the efficacy of indigenous healing compare with that of professional clinical care, and what does it tell us about the nature of the healing process? Can we learn anything practically useful, either to solve problems besetting contemporary health care or for treating sickness in different societies (Kleinman and Sung 1979; Subedi 2001)?

Traditional medicine has a long history, it is the "sum total of the knowledge, skills and practices based on theories, beliefs and experiences indigenous to different cultures whether explicable or not, used in the maintenance of health as well as in the prevention, diagnosis, improvement or treatment of physical and mental illness" (WHO 2013: 15). Across the world traditional medicine is the major health care system or serves as a complement to modern medicine. Many scholars use traditional medicine, indigenous medicine, and complementary medicine interchangeably. For many people in lower-income countries like Nepal, herbal medicine, traditional treatments, and traditional practitioners are the main health care providers. In general such services are close to home, culturally acceptable and trusted by a large number of people, easily accessible, and affordable.

A traditional healer or practitioner is a person who is recognized by the community in which he/she lives as competent to provide health care by using vegetable, animal, and mineral substances and other methods based on the knowledge, attitudes and beliefs that are prevalent in the community regarding physical, mental, and social well-being, and of the causes for diseases and disability (Kristvik 1999). According to the WHO, at least 80 percent of the population in developing countries relies entirely on the traditional healing systems as their primary health care service (Bodeker 1997 quoted in Tamang et al. 2001).

Even such a broad definition, however, does not capture the tremendous variety of traditional health care either within or among countries. In the west, the most influential version of healing was the humoral medicine of classic Greece, where the body–mind entity was viewed as consisting of earth, water, fire, and air, each with its associated sensory qualities (e.g. wetness and hotness) which are supposed to be in a specific balance for each individual (Logan 1977). Illness is identified as an excess of any of these components and, therefore, treated through increasing or reducing their presence. Hence a diagnosed excess of fire associated with the humor yellow bile was treated through the addition of water or appropriately cold foods; and excess of air associated with the humor blood through bleeding, and so on (Doyal 1987). Not only did this become the foundation for medieval and European medicine until the 19th century, it is still practiced as Unani medicine in Islamic countries. In parts of Latin America humoral medicine has a close resemblance to Ayurvedic medicine in India and Nepal. In China and India, ancient traditions of Chinese medicine and Indian Ayurvedic medicine are taught and practiced in medical schools and institutions. Other countries in Asia, such as Vietnam and the Philippines, have developed their own systems of indigenous health care by borrowing extensively from Chinese traditional medicine. Such coherent and institutionalized traditions are found primarily in Asia.

The concept of Yin and Yang bears a close resemblance to the Greek thinking that there must be a balance between the naturally recuperative powers of the body, and that specific techniques can be used to restore this balance. The use of acupuncture, along with its associated ideas of meridians, is unique to the Chinese tradition. The curative and explanatory aims of both are still based on the belief that the health of each individual depends upon obtaining equilibrium between the internal components and external influences that either maintain or disrupt this equilibrium. It is now accepted in both western and eastern countries that acupuncture is effective for treating a variety of illnesses involving chronic pain that are untreatable by conventional means (Doyal 1987).

As long as such systems of healing provide internally consistent experiences of health, illness, and healing, why should they not be endorsed as at least equal partners with the biomedical approach in tackling the health problems of populations in which they are already a part? As three former executives of WHO put it (quoted in Doyal 1987: 30): "The fact [is] that there are very few places in the world where traditional healers are not practicing. . . . Traditional healers are dealing more or less satisfactorily with many of the health problems of the local people."

Reliable data on the extent of indigenous health care practices and the number of traditional practitioners are not available. Information obtained from surveys is thought to underestimate the importance of traditional medicine because respondents are reluctant to reveal the extent of their reliance on traditional care to researchers who generally have a modern perspective. In addition, health surveys fail to capture rare and seasonal events because they use short recall periods in order to increase the responses' reliability.

Traditional health care practices in Nepal

Traditional health care in Nepal includes a wide variety of practices carried out by *Jari buti wala* or *Vaidya* (herbalists), *Sudheni* (birth attendants), *Dhami, Jhankri, Janne Manchhe*, and faith healers and diviners, depending on their own worldview (Subedi 2001). Tremendous ethnic diversity contributes to further variation in healing practices. Moreover, many indigenous Nepali healers combine modern health care technologies with traditional practices, making the modifier 'traditional' somewhat inappropriate. Because of the heterogeneity and fluidity of indigenous health care in Nepal, one must carefully avoid generalizations.

Information on Nepal's rich heritage of indigenous health care can be drawn primarily from ethnographic studies of healers in particular communities. Traditional medicine has been widely practiced in Nepal from time immemorial, providing a wide range of preventive, promotional, curative, and rehabilitating services. After the introduction of the biomedicine system, the Government of Nepal has accepted the following four formal traditions of medicine: Allopathic, Ayurvedic, natural therapy, and the Unani tradition.

In Chapter 2, "Healer Choice in Medically Pluralistic Cultural Settings," Ayurveda was said to be a part of the national health system in

Nepal under the MoHP. Many Ayurvedic medical shops are providing medical treatment in Nepal. At least four types of Ayurvedic practitioners are working in Nepal: those who are not institutionally trained but gained knowledge through their family traditions; the herbalists who practice with local medicinal plants; institutionally qualified Ayurvedic health professionals; and the graduates of Allopathic medicine who trust Ayurveda as a supplementary option. All of them emphasize Ayurveda's preventive and promoting aspects, focusing on food habits, personal hygiene, and social behavior. People in Nepal believe that Ayurvedic medicines do not have side effects.

Acupuncture, the traditional Chinese medicine or 'needle therapy', is also common in Nepal. The concept of Yin and Yang is fundamental for understanding acupuncture. A person is considered as a microcosm in the universe and a healthy body requires a balance between the forces of Yin and Yang. Acupuncture's theoretical basis is that there are patterns of *qi* that flows through the pathways-meridians of the body, and any potential disruptions of this *qi* flows are believed to be responsible for diseases (Subedi 2001). Acupuncture treatment can correct imbalances in the flow of *qi* by inserting a needle at identified acupuncture points.

Homeopathy, introduced in Nepal during the 1920s, is a therapeutic natural healing. Today, there is one Homeopathy hospital, and a government Unani dispensary in Kathmandu. *Amchi*, the Tibetan system of medicine is practiced in the upper Himalayan regions. In addition, there are traditional healers who, normally being local persons, tend to reflect local customs and beliefs, often being the principal health care providers in the villages. They deal with physical and mental ailments by prayers, sacred axioms, amulets, herbs, barks, mysticisms, etc.

Until recently, traditional practitioners provided the only health care accessible to the majority of the population in Nepal. Even today, allopathic medical services do not reach many rural areas. For instance, Mohin Shah (1977: 31) stated that, in the Tanahu district, the government health services in the late 1970s provided barely 10 percent of all consultations by people seeking health care, and that they took care of only 3 percent of ill persons' estimated needs. One study (Shrestha and Lediard 1980) estimated that, in 1978–1979, there were four to eight hundred thousand faith healers in Nepal, and about 500 doctors and 1,500 paramedics. According to the 1998 Nepal Human Development Report, only 10 percent of the total population of Nepal had access to government-provided formal health services (NESAC 1998). Even after putting in a great deal of resources and efforts, the health services provided by the government reached no more than 40 percent of the population in 2015.

One of the biggest challenges in the public health sector in Nepal is the inefficient information and management system, and the data are not reliable (Ministry of Health 1999). The recruitment and deployment of health workforce in the public sector is a long and complicated process that involves multiple agencies and political interests among the power elites. The coordination between the Ministry of Education and Ministry of Health is poor for the production and recruitment of the health workforce.

Growing recognition of traditional health care

Before 1950, government clinics and hospitals in Nepal provided health care to government officials and a small elite living in urban areas (Dixit 1999; Subedi 2001). For centuries, indigenous healers and traditional practitioners were the only health workers available for people in general, and for those living in rural areas in particular. There are several reasons for justifying the use of traditional, indigenous health care in Nepal and to accept that traditional practitioners can coexist with the allopathic medicine (Justice 1986; Dixit 1999; Subedi 2001): its intrinsic medical relevance, people's faith in and access to different health care providers, and the government's health policy.

Herbal medicines are used in Nepal for different purposes. For example, in the correct combinations and amounts, they have shown to be effective for treating high blood pressure, digestive problems, and arthritis. Historically, the medical uses of herbs were explored in different cultures as a part of folk healing traditions.

The reality even now is that a large proportion of the rural population visits traditional healers before they seek government-provided services or private practitioners of Allopathic medicine. First, patients feel comfortable with traditional healers who reside in the community and are familiar with the social context. Modern health care workers, in contrast, may be regarded as outsiders. Second, patients are frequently dissatisfied with the quality of modern health care because health care providers are often perceived as unsympathetic and unresponsive to the patient's concerns and needs. Third, traditional health services are usually more accessible than modern health care. They are not far away from home and people do not have to spend money to travel to the modern health care centers. Fourth, many people's preference for traditional health care also reflects the fact that traditional medicines consist of substances or instruments that are grown or produced indigenously and, therefore, by and large are much cheaper than allopathic medicines. Besides, paying for traditional medicine can be done, for instance, in kind, offering gifts at a later time, or even by negotiating the amount. Fifth, traditional healers treat diseases holistically, often including the patient's family, even the community, in the treatment. Many people also believe that the side effects of traditional medicine (especially herbal medicine, physiotherapy, and psychosomatic healing) are fewer compared to allopathic medicine.

The increased interest in traditional health care is due to the fact that it has become more obvious that modern health services have not gained full confidence among the people they have set out to serve. Many patients have expressed concern regarding the poor quality of care rendered by modern health care institutions. Patients frequently have objected to the failure of modern medicine to address their problems in a holistic manner (Heggenhougen 1987). In general, a pattern seems to emerge whereby patients tend to consult modern health care services for infectious diseases for which modern health care has proved to be highly effective (Subedi 2001), while other diseases remain within the domain of traditional medicine: chronic conditions, complaints related to psychological or social disruptions, problems associated with reproductions (e.g. infertility, menstrual disorders), diseases caused by organisms which have become resistant to drugs, and diseases that respond slowly to biomedical treatments.

The Government of Nepal has not formally recognized the indigenous healing system and the healers as partners in the country's formal health care system. Neither are there any concrete government policy and programs designed to appreciate, encourage, and develop this informal healing system being managed by traditional practitioners all over the country (Tamang et al. 2001). The fact is that there are large numbers of personnel who, if properly used, can be a great force for education and change in matters concerning health (Dixit 1999). However, some research and training has been done for using them in health education, family planning, and treatment of diarrhea (SCF-UK 1997). Also, some nongovernment organizations have involved traditional practitioners in programs for family planning awareness, immunization and diarrhea control, but not really appreciating their knowledge and healing system as equal partners (Tamang et al. 2001).

Many observers now recognize that traditional practitioners provide valuable health care and that supplementing their training would enable them to meet many health needs. The interest increased notably after the notion of primary health care became a key issue in the late 1970s, exemplified with the 1977 Alma Ata Declaration on Primary Health Care (WHO 1978), which emphasized the importance of utilizing existing resources fully and relying on the community in order to meet health care needs.

Although surveys provide only a snapshot of the traditional healers' numbers and activities, it seems clear that a substantial proportion of ill people consult traditional healers in Nepal. Many traditional practitioners are old, and their number is declining in rural areas due to impact of westernization and modernization. The declining prestige and credibility of traditional healers, which has resulted from modernization, is also making it difficult to find replacements.

Traditional health care is unlikely to disappear, particularly if the quality of, and access to, modern health care service does not improve significantly. The boundaries between traditional and modern health care practitioners are beginning to blur, with the former adopting many of the latter's practices. The competition between the two groups will likely necessitate a health care policy that addresses the entire spectrum of health care, traditional and modern, and the relationship between them.

Traditional medical practice in Nepal is changing in response also to social and economic developments. For example, economic modernization has affected the way in which many traditional practitioners operate, for instance, prescribing antibiotics, dressing in white coats, and operating from modern clinical facilities. Their clinics have waiting rooms, and they use stethoscopes and keep record cards. These developments reflect not only increasing competition with modern health care providers, but also changes in the contents of traditional health care. Traditional practitioners are also becoming increasingly professionalized and specialized, even referring cases to each other.

Possible policy options

Recently, India, China, and other Asian countries have begun to integrate indigenous medicine with modern health care. For example, in China 'barefoot doctors' were recruited from the rank of traditional herbalists to become the keystone of China's primary health care system. The Chinese have reported dramatic improvements in the health conditions following the incorporation of traditional health workers into the modern system. Many primary health care systems have trained and employed traditional birth attendants (TBA) to provide modern antenatal and postnatal care, particularly in rural communities. TBA training programs in Brazil, Thailand, and several African countries, like Sudan, Zimbabwe, Tanzania, and Ethiopia, have demonstrated that TBAs can contribute successfully to primary health care programs (Dejong 1991). These experiments also have suggested the possibility that other traditional healers, such as bonesetters and traditional dentists, might be involved more fully in the provision of modern health care (Dejong 1991). Also the WHO has encouraged an increased use of indigenous medicine.

Despite many countries and WHO having acknowledged the value of indigenous medicine, the Government of Nepal has been reluctant to formally recognize traditional medicine. The following discussion reviews some of the possible public policy options with regard to traditional healers.

By ignoring traditional health care, the government has left traditional healers unrecognized, unregulated, and free to respond in various ways to demands for their services. This strategy clearly makes it impossible for the government to supervise the training of traditional health workers or regulate traditional health practices. It also hinders the possibility of including traditional medicine in a national health plan for developing health personnel and service expansion. Moreover, ignoring traditional medicine prevents the exchange of information between modern health care workers and traditional practitioners. Reliance on traditional treatment may delay the use of modern health care where it would be more appropriate, resulting in diseases progressing beyond the stage where it can be treated effectively.

If we do not adopt policies with regard to traditional health care, we reduce our opportunity to learn about its pharmacopoeia, and to discourage the use of those substances that are harmful and promoting those that are valuable (Unschuld 1976). Some traditional remedies are clearly beneficial. For example, scientists have identified active ingredients including anti-hypertension, or inflammation reduction agents, which alleviate spasms and asthma. On the other hand, some practices are harmful. For example, traditional birth attendants are known to use oxytocin substances for women who have a hemorrhage during labor or delivery.

Biomedical practitioners undergo standardized training before they enter the profession. This provides opportunities to instill codes of professional conduct and to ensure that minimum qualifications are fulfilled. In contrast, traditional practitioners in Nepal are highly heterogeneous; they do not subscribe to a common ethics code or undergo a prescribed program of preparation. Professional associations of traditional practitioners might be encouraged to serve these two important functions.

Licensing is a form of official, selective recognition that enables to restrict the number of entrants into the profession and to define their qualifications. This approach has strong advantages. First, licensing may serve as a mechanism for encouraging traditional healers to increase their technical knowledge and to establish minimum standards of training. Second, it may help to open official channels of communication between the two parallel health care systems. Third, it may encourage modern health care practitioners to learn about the wider range of factors that can be considered when diagnosing and treating patient. The magnitude of benefits from licensing depends on the competence and integrity of the licensing authority, and criteria adopted for conferring licenses.

The professional associations also provide a mechanism for promoting their members' interests and for enhancing their political authority when informing government agencies and the public in general about traditional health care.

The government may promote traditional health care by granting some kind of subsidies. Authorities can provide adequate supplies of drugs and other material for free or at reduced prices. Similarly, government agencies can offer training opportunities such as short, flexible courses in modern diagnostic and treatment techniques. Selective subsidizing is also a way to encourage those healers who meet certain established criteria, such as completing training courses. Evidence suggests that at least for traditional birth attendants, modest training in aseptic techniques and the recognition of certain symptoms or complication substantially increase the value of some traditional treatment and strengthen the services that these practitioners provide.

Training traditional birth attendants to provide prenatal and postnatal care, to perform safe deliveries, and to refer obstetric emergencies is perhaps the area of greatest potential payoff in linking traditional and modern health care. Traditional birth attendants are more likely than modern sector health care providers to be well known to the patient, and to offer continuous care in the community, before, during, and after child birth.

Training objectives should be modest and very clear. They might include, for example, encouraging women to speak about prenatal care, identifying high risk women and referring them to specialists, teaching traditional birth attendants to reduce the risks of infection or trauma (e.g. discouraging the inappropriate use of herbs or unsterilized instruments on the umbilical cord), and encouraging women to use family planning after delivery.

Enforcement of these rules and regulations has to be carried out at the district or local level in order to ensure continuity and to allow for variations in local conditions and practices. The diversity in types of healers suggests a need for public policies tailored to the constraints and opportunities of each type of traditional practitioners. These local ideas and practices would be references for other health workers and agents responsible for change, for instance, in health education. Such beliefs, ideas, and practices make sense to the local people.

Despite these obvious advantages, traditional healing can serve to obscure the real causes of diseases, standing in the way of the accurate medical understanding and political struggle necessary to eliminate them. This means that national health strategies should focus on prevention rather than cure, and on political and economic strategies to shape and mold the environment accordingly. This is why WHO policies on traditional healing rightly focus on the retraining of traditional healers in primary health care rather than on an uncritical acceptance of various belief systems. Dubos (1980: 427), for example, rightly says:

> on the one hand, science can eventually solve the technical aspects of almost any medical problem. On the other hand, the application of medical knowledge to the prevention and treatment of disease will be necessarily limited by economic and other social factors. Choices have to be made among all the possibilities for medical care and disease prevention, but there is no agreement as to the social or ethical bases on which to make choices.

The importance given to a particular disease or group of diseases, differs from one culture or one social group to another, and furthermore changes with time. The principal objective of a national health policy must be to upgrade the health standards of the majority of the population by strengthening the primary health care system, making effective health care services readily available at the local level; extending basic primary health services to the village level and providing the rural population with the benefits of modern medical facilities and trained health care providers by developing different existing health care traditions in Nepal. Based on a country's realities, models for integrating traditional medicine into the national health system should be explored. The goal should be to develop models for health care delivery which are sustainable and feasible, and which will improve health outcomes. The traditional systems of healing have much to contribute to solve the health problems of developing countries like Nepal.

Note

1 A version of this chapter originally appeared as 'Indigenous Knowledge and Health Development in Nepal: An Anthropological Inquiry', *Manav Samaj*, 1: 135–151, 2004. Used with permission.

References

Dejong, Jocelyn. 1991. *Traditional Medicine in Sub-Saharan Africa.* Policy Research and External Affairs, Population and Human Resources Department, the World Bank.

Dixit, Hemang. 1999. *The Quest for Health* (2nd Edition). Kathmandu: Educational Enterprise (P) Ltd.

Doyal, Len. 1987. "Health, Underdevelopment and Traditional Medicine." *Holistic Medicine* 2: 27–40.

Dubos, Rene. 1980. *Man Adapting.* New Haven and London: Yale University Press.

Gill, Gerald J. 1993. "Indigenous System in Agriculture and Resource Management: An Overview." In D. Tamang, G. J. Gill and G. B. Thapa, eds., *Indigenous Management of Natural Resources in Nepal*, pp. 3–12. Kathmandu: HMG, MoA and Winrock International.

Gillam, Stephen. 1989. "The Traditional Healers as Village Health Worker." *Journal of Institute of Medicine* 11: 67–76.

Heggenhougen, H. K. 1987. "Traditional Medicine in Developing Countries: Intrinsic Value and Relevance for Holistic Health Care." *Holistic Medicine* 2: 47–56.

IIRR. 1996. *Recording and Using Indigenous Knowledge: A Manual.* Silang, Cavite, Philippines: International Institute of Rural Reconstruction.

Justice, Judith. 1986. *Policies, Plans & People: Foreign Aid and Health Development.* Berkeley: University of California Press.

Kamanta, Yoji. 2000. "Indigenous Knowledge, Cultural Empowerment and Alternatives." *Contributions to Nepalese Studies* 27(1): 51–69. CNAS, TU.

Kleinman, Arthur and Lilias H. Sung. 1979. "Why Do Indigenous Practitioners Successfully Heal?" *Social Science and Medicine* 13B: 7–26.

Kristvik, Ellen. 1999. *Drums and Syringes.* Bibliotheca Himalayica Series III, Vol. 7, Kathmandu: EMR.

Logan, Michael H. 1977. "Anthropological Research on the Hot-Cold Theory of Disease: Some Methodological Suggestions." *Medical Anthropology* 1(4).

Ministry of Health. 1999. *Second Long-Term Health Plan (1997–2017).* Kathmandu: HMG and Ministry of Health.

NESAC. 1998. *Nepal Human Development Report 1998.* Kathmandu: NESAC.

Save the Children. 1997. *Traditional Healers and Health Post Peons as Alternative Health Care Providers: Experiences of SCF (UK) Nepal.* Kathmandu: Save the Children.

Shah, Moin. 1977. *Rural Health Needs: Report of a Study in the Primary Health Care Unit (District) of Tanahu, Nepal.* Maharajgunj, Kathmandu: Institute of Medicine, Health Manpower Development Research Project.

Shrestha, Ramesh M. and Mark Lediard. 1980. *Faith Healers: A Force for Change.* Kathmandu: Project Supported by UNFPA, Published with UNICEF Assistance.

Subedi, Madhusudan Sharma. 2001. *Medical Anthropology of Nepal.* Kathmandu: Udaya Books.

Tamang, Parshuram et al. 2001. *Tamang Healing in the Himalaya: A Study on the Tamang Healing Knowledge and the Development Interventions in and around Langtang National Park of Central Nepal.* Kathmandu: Milijuli.

Unschuld, Paul U. 1976. "Western Medicine and Traditional Healing System: Competition, Cooperation or Integration?" In *Ethics in Science and Medicine* Vol. 3, pp. 1–20. Great Britain: Pergamon Press.

WHO. 2013. *WHO Traditional Medicine Strategy 2014–2013.* Geneva: WHO.

WHO. 1978. *Declaration of Alma-Ata.* Geneva: WHO.

5 Food, health, and illness ideology in Kirtipur[1]

Food is one of the major topics of common interest among both the health professions and the social sciences. From the dawn of medical history the role of food in health and for explaining diseases has been under investigation by health workers, and its significance increases as further advances in nutritional knowledge are made (Cassel 1977). In medical anthropology the study of food ways and the set of attitudes, beliefs, and practices surrounding food is one important way to unravel the complexities of a community's overall cultural pattern (Caplan 1997; Good 1994; Lowdin 1985; Subedi 2001).

In this chapter I argue that the principles underlying food classification and its relation to health and illness are playing an important role for people's use and non-use of particular food to maintain good health. Finally, the categories, beliefs, and practices concerning food should be seen as tools for understanding and explaining people's strategies to cope with illness.

Material and methods

The research for this chapter was designed to explore any systematic relationship between food categories and people's help-seeking behavior when they experienced various types of illnesses. In July–December 1999 I collected information by interviewing people in Kirtipur, a Newari town in the Kathmandu Valley.

My sample consisted of males and females, educated and uneducated, patients and healers, and the interviews were done both individually and collectively. The discussions about food types, beliefs, and the use of food as part of an illness ideology were unstructured and in-depth and sometimes lasted for more than two hours. Some of the informants were confused and did not have concrete ideas about the types of food, while other informants had contradictory views of the classification of foods, with or without reasoning.

I argue that the reality can only be fully understood by examining the specific cultural contexts and the dominant worldview among people. As Kleinman (1978, 1980) pointed out, individuals are more likely to have quite vague and indefinite models for explaining their illness, depending on past experiences and his/her circle of kin and friends. This tendency in research, in my view, is equally applicable to understand the way people think about food and illness.

Results and discussion

Conceptualizing food and food classification

Food is more than just a source of nutrition. People do not eat protein and carbohydrates, but just food. Nutritional anthropologists and medical anthropologists are concerned with the symbolic meaning of food in different cultures, and with the ways in which types of food are combined to form culturally acceptable meals. In all human societies, food plays many roles, and is deeply embedded in the social, religious, and economic aspects of everyday life. It also carries with it a range of social and symbolic meanings both expressing and creating meaning between human beings and deities, and the natural environment. In other words, food is never 'just food', and its significance is more than nutritional. It is intimately bound up with social relations, cultural ideas, and economic status (Caplan 1997; Geertz 1973; Good 1994; Helman 1996; Lowdin 1985; McElroy and Townsend 1996). The individual, the family, and the wider social network play a decisive part in shaping the willingness and ability of a person to change his/her food choices. The transformation of 'raw' into 'cooked' food is one of the defining features of human societies, a key criterion of 'culture' as opposed to 'nature' (Chowdhury et al. 2000).

In Nepal, households select and consume food within the constraints of *jat* (caste) restrictions. Primary and essential means of classifying food relate to their purity. Higher *jat* or *jatis* people must avoid polluting types of food to retain their *jat* status, while lower *jatis* are permitted to consume many of the polluting types of food. I equate this classification of the degree of polluted food with the *triguna* food classification mentioned in the literature (Pool 1987; Chowdhury et al. 2000; Subedi 2001). According to a Brahman pandit in Kirtipur, there are three categories of food: *satavik*, *rajasa*, and *tamasa*. *Satavik* food is 'cool', including sacred food such as milk, *ghieu* (butter), most fruits, and vegetables. The *satavik* diet is strictly vegetarian, and also regards certain vegetables like onion and garlic as impure. These types of food generate goodness and joy and inspire all novel virtues and actions. *Rajasa* food is 'hot', and includes meat, eggs, onions, and garlic. These types of food produce egoism, selfishness, violence, jealousy, and ambition. *Rajasa* food is for the kings and warriors. *Tamas* are spoiled and stale beef and alcohol, and permit all the items in the two previous categories. These types of food are linked to stupidity, laziness, fear, and all sorts of basic behavior. *Tamasic* food is for demons. The underlying conception is that food determines men's mood and actions. Under the traditional ideology, Brahmins have a *satagun* temperament, and should consume *satavik* food only; Chhetries have *rajogun* temperament, and should consume *rajasa* and *satavik* food; Sudra have *tamogun* temperament, and are permitted to consume *tamas* food as well as the other two types.

Although, people talk about *satavik, rajasik,* and *tamasik* food in Kirtipur, the empirical evidences of these criteria for the differentiation of food, and who should eat which categories of food, seems rare. Contrary to this classical food categorization, animal sacrifice, meat consumption, and drinking alcoholic beverages are culturally prescribed in a Newari cultural context. I have some trouble explaining why or how the flesh of a buffalo or pig is more polluting than that of goat or chicken. One Brahmin felt it was because pigs and water buffaloes eat feces but goats do not. Other respondents, however, noted that goats also eat feces. Whatever the reason, chicken and especially goats are viewed as purer than pigs or water buffaloes. Thus, I can clearly say that the classification of food into *Satavik, Rajasa,* and *Tamas* may have been written in some religious texts, a line of reasoning not practiced by people.

The widespread ethno-medical system is an equilibrium model. Food, vegetables, and drinks are marked by unchanging hot and cold metaphorical qualities. Health is thought to depend on maintaining the body's temperature balance, an equilibrium constantly threatened by the metaphorical and thermal forces to which it is exposed (Foster 1994). An excess of metaphorical and thermal hot and cold leads to illness, thus, hot is a remedy for cold illnesses and cold is a remedy for hot illnesses. This ethno-medical system is widely known as the 'hot–cold' balance. The division of food into hot and cold is a feature of many cultural groups in the Islamic world, the Indian sub-continent, Latin America, and China (Foster 1994; Pool 1987). In all these cultures, the binary system of classification includes much more than food: medicines, illnesses, mental and physical states, and natural and supernatural forces are all grouped into either hot or cold categories (Foster 1994; Helman 1996; Pool 1987; Subedi 2001).

The notion of hot and cold does not usually refer only to actual temperatures, but rather to certain symbolic values associated with each category of foodstuff. The words *garmi* (hot) and *thandi* or *sardi* (cold) when used in connection with food refer to a number of qualities. First, *tato* (hot) and *chiso* (cold) refer to temperature. *Khana dherai tato chha, kehi samaya pachhi khane* ("the food is very hot, could you please wait for a moment before eating it") is a common expression in Nepal to indicate the thermal condition of the food. Similarly, they say, "this food is *chiso* (cold), please heat it before you eat." Second, they refer to abstract qualities, which usually bear no relation to temperature. All types of food, all herbal and other remedies, weather and timing during the day or the year, have a hot or cold value that all have to harmonize to avoid problems. Health is defined as a balance between these categories and classified into hot and cold affiliations.

People also think about the bodily constitution in terms of hot and cold. A person with a hot constitution is thought to be more prone to a hot disease than a person with a cold constitution and vice versa. A person with a cold constitution may eat as much hot food as he/she likes without contracting a hot disease, and a person with a hot constitution is less likely to get a cold disease from eating cold food. This can only be discovered empirically after some years of experience have shown to which disease a person is prone. For example, if the parents notice that, after the family has eaten hot food, one of their children repeatedly comes out with a rash (a hot disease), while the others do not, and this appears to occur more frequently during the summer, they will conclude that the child has a hot constitution. Another example is if a woman has had three or four spontaneous miscarriages (caused by too much heat), then her relatives will consider this to be proof that she has a hot constitution. Therefore, they will make sure that she avoids hot types of food during subsequent pregnancies. Thus a hot constitution appears to mean the same as being prone to hot diseases and a cold constitution to cold diseases.

The constitution is also seen as being related to personality traits. For example, people with hot constitutions are more likely to be hot tempered, whereas those with cold constitutions are more likely to be mild tempered. Diet, in conjunction with a specific constitution, can also influence the temperament. For some informants in Kirtipur, this was how they explained why people who drink excessively are bad tempered and aggressive. Alcohol is hot, and if a person with an already hot constitution drinks a lot, then the amount of heat in that person's body will become so great that he/she will become angry and aggressive.

In addition, environmental conditions such as seasonal temperature variations and exposure to the hot sun may affect people's health, especially if the person concerned has a hot constitution or has been eating hot types of food. During the winter people are more prone to have cold diseases and will therefore try to avoid cold types of food.

Perceptions of food and health in Kirtipur

Keeping a balance between *garmi* (hot) and *sardi* or *thandi* (cold) is crucial for maintaining good health in Nepal. The notion of a balance between hot and cold is a basic principle in the classical Hindu medicine, Ayurveda, and also in Tibetan medicine, both of which have influenced Nepali ways of thinking about illness and health. The hot–cold principle leads to continuous attempts at re-establishing the critical balance between opposite forces, in themselves not good or bad, but dangerous if reaching extremes.

In order to strike the right balance, people in Kirtipur treat a particular illness by adding hot or cold types of food or medicine to the diet. One of the most common questions a patient or the relative of the patient asks any practitioner during the consultation is what types of food should and should not be consumed. The question refers to the patient's illness as well as to the type of medication administered by the practitioners. Each sick person or his/her relative expects that a practitioner will offer advice about the diet after considering the illness, the patient's body constitution, and the quality of medicine administered. Food is thought to enhance and facilitate the effects of the medicines, and to provide a means of balancing the extreme qualities of medicines.

The concept of a balance between hot and cold has led to a vast number of rules for daily life, including what, how, and when to eat. All kinds of food are classified with regard to heating and cooking capacities. When there is disequilibrium between hot and cold, a cold condition needs to be heated up, and a hot condition needs cooling down. Such adjustment attempts are among the main health care measures taken within the popular health care sectors. Taking hot types of food during the hot condition and cold types of food during the cold condition are perceived as dangerous. People in Kirtipur also related hot and cold to other sources, such as physical labor and sexual intercourse. Pregnant women are advised to refrain from heavy work because increased body heat may lead to a miscarriage. Sex is generally considered to be hot or heat producing. Engaging in sexual intercourse while in a state of fever is considered particularly dangerous, and quite possibly fatal. One informant suggested this act as a cause of typhoid.

Perceiving that having sexual intercourse simultaneously with having a fever may be based on a notion of illness deriving from excessive or unbalanced 'hotness', that is, both the fever and the sexual activity produce too much heat in the body.

If the symptoms of illness appear, the first measures are taken at home. The first task is one of interpretation by trying to discern what kind of ailment one is dealing with. Coughing will tend to be understood as a cold condition that needs to be regulated. Attempts to adjust the hot–cold balance in the body are mainly done by diet. For a cold condition, cold food like fruits and curd are to be avoided. But it is not always as straightforward as that. Sometimes, even a condition that is judged as hot, like fever, can call for hot types of food, and a high intake of hot types of food can then be taken to heat up the body even further. The guiding principle here is bringing the heat to a maximum so that it can subside again.

People in Kirtipur could not differentiate some of the food into two extreme valences and categorized them as neither *sardi* nor *garmi* (neutral or intermediate). This type of food classification is common throughout Nepal (Blustain 1976; Stone 1976). Almost all food, according to local classification in Kirtipur, can be assigned to one of three categories, *garmi* (hot), *sardi* (cold), or neither *garmi* nor *sardi* (neutral or intermediate).

When I understood that people in Kirtipur classified food into these three different categories based on their own ideas, I asked them to classify locally available food into these categories. This task was not easy, however, and the criteria reported varied. Sometimes they disagreed with one another and tried to give their own reasons. Table 5.1 shows a simplified classification of locally available food in Kirtipur.

Table 5.1 Hot, neutral, and cold classification of locally available food in Kirtipur

Hot types of foods (*Garmi khana*)	Breast milk, Just boiled dairy milk, Goat meat, Soybeans, *Ghieu* (butter), Peanuts, Garlic, Pepper, Tea, *Raksi* (homemade liquor), Coffee, Mustard oil, *Jwano* soup, Meat *Masala* and Garam *Masala* (spices in general), Local chicken, Tobacco, Cumin, Ginger, Honey, Walnut, Wheat, *Gahat* (Horse gram)
Neutral food (*Na garmi na sardi*)	Onion, Eggs, Milk (cow), Mango, Buffalo meat, Rice, Carrot, Lemon, Bitten rice, Kidney beans, Dried beans, Broiler, Lady's finger, Mushroom, *Karela* (bitter melon), *Palungi* (Spinach), Papaya
Cold types of foods (*Sardi Khana*)	Cauliflower, Cabbage, *Tama* (bamboo-shoots), Green cucumber, Pumpkin, Orange, Apple, Yogurt, Banana, Tomato, Green-leaf vegetables, Green beans, Radish, Pork, Sugarcane, Guava, Coca Cola

In most cases, these food classifications were not based on logically consistent principles. Food classified as hot in one culture, area or region, are not necessarily seen as hot in another (Foster 1994). The hot–cold value of meat varied, for example, though people spoke of meat in general as hot. Buffalo meat was seen as relatively cold. All informants categorized local chicken as very hot. Goat meat was not considered as hot as local chicken (or chicken in general), but hotter than buffalo meat. Interestingly, pork meat was considered to be cold, while goat and chicken meat were considered hot, contrary to what might be expected using the *triguna* system. Most fruit and vegetables tended to be considered neutral or cold. Grain showed a wide diversity: rice was neutral, rice fried in *ghieu* (butter) was considered hot, and wheat was considered hot.

There were many individual variations in Kirtipur with regard to many types of food being hot, neutral, and cold. There were significant disagreements regarding the hot–cold classifications, contrasting with Blustain's (1976) work in an ethnically diverse village in the Gorkha district. She found almost a universal agreement among independently interviewed informants on which types of food belonged to each category. Why was there a disagreement in my study? First, because I was working in an area dominated by a Newari population among an ethnically diverse population. Second, many informants explained that cold or hot types of food were seen as causing illness, and people tended to classify food they felt made them sick as cold or hot. Third, in the average people's mind, most food may not be clearly classified – many people may simply have guessed.

When asked to tell why certain types of food were *garmi* or *sardi*, most informants' standard answer was, "because it is" or "I think it is" or "in my view . . . mm." or "well, it is because it works." Nor could they explain why, for example, local chicken should be hot, but broiler should be neutral. Most people usually attempt to interpret causes of a specific illness and find it difficult to think about this in more general terms. Therefore, to relate illness to types of food appears to be used as a post-hoc explanation, especially when an individual is already ill. The hot–cold distinction of food is more salient when a person is in vulnerable states, such as pregnancy or postpartum period. Lactating mothers told me that their diet should be modified according to the general health of the infant receiving breast milk. If the baby had a cold category illness, she avoided cold types of food that might turn the breast cold and thus aggravate the illness.

If the qualities of hot and cold are not based on the thermal temperature and food is categorized on the basis of their intrinsic properties, how then do people know whether a particular type of food is hot or cold? The informants' general answer was that they deduced the quality of the food from the effect it was supposed to have on the person who ate it. For example, one informant said, "bananas are cold because eating too much bananas in the cold season causes cough and cold (which are cold diseases)." This season-related practice of hot/cold avoidance appeared to be more important when individuals were perceived as being in a vulnerable state.

In Kirtipur, many community members classified food in terms of digestibility. Food being difficult to digest were said to make one sick, especially with diarrhea, vomiting, or a cold. One Brahmin woman remarked:

> Easy-to-digest types of food are rice, bread and lentil. It depends on the season; in the summer season it is hard to digest new wheat bread. It also depends on how much you eat. If you eat lightly, it is easy to digest. Rice makes the stomach big (*bhudi badhau chha*), it is easy to digest, but it is not as strengthening as bread. Meat is difficult to digest. You should eat *supari* (betal nut), or *dahi* (yogurt) and/or sweets afterwards, or best eat yogurt. You should eat equally, but light in the morning and heavy in the evening.

Digestibility is particularly important within different age groups. Young children and elderly both require easily digestible food. In general poorly cooked food and fat meat is considered hard to digest. Many kinds of legumes, such as soybeans, peanuts, and *gahat* (horse gram) are considered hard to digest, especially for people in vulnerable phases of life or in particular states (such as infancy or postpartum). However, digestibility did not appear to be related to the hot–cold characteristics of food. For instance, chicken and goat meat were considered to be hot food, but chicken was seen as easy to digest, while goat meat was difficult to digest.

Food is often classified by taste. In general, Nepali food has strong flavors: sweet, salty, sour, and spicy. Food without salt or spices or bitter food was not popular in Kirtipur. Bitter is the taste of medicine (*Ausadhi khayako jasto*), that is, as if taking medicine. Taste is linked with the food-related treatment of illness. Sour, hot, and spicy food was not given to children with cough and colds. One of my informants stated that when someone has a cold or cough, sweet food (such as banana, ice cream, honey, sugar, and different types of sweets) should be avoided, and hot water or bitter food (boiled water mixed with turmeric powder, hot lemon) is especially important. For fever, spicy food and chilies should be avoided as they all have heating properties.

People perceive certain types of food as being beneficial for their health. Most people living in Kirtipur considered animal products like milk, meat, *ghieu* (butter), *dahi* (yogurt), and eggs as healthy. The notion of healthiness of particular types of food is related in part to a notion of the *tagatilo* (nutrient or having vitamins). I spoke with several men and women about *tagatilo* food and vitamins: what they were, where they were found, and what they did? One of my informants gave her opinion of *tagatilo* food:

> *Tagatilo* food or vitamins give you strength and make you healthy. They are found in all food: apples, oranges, bananas, milk, yogurt, soybeans, green vegetables . . . all food. All our homegrown food has vitamins, but if we buy old food from the *bazaar* (market) they hardly have vitamins left. Vitamins make you healthy and reduce diseases and kill all types of parasites. Vitamins are not the same as medicine. Medicines are for diseases, and vitamins to keep the body strong and healthy.

The view expressed clearly raises the question about the quality of food in the market. When a woman was asked why homegrown food has vitamins and food from the market have hardly any vitamins left, she replied:

> Everybody knows about it. Most of the food at the market comes from the Tarai and India. Nobody cares about it. I have not heard about the quality control mechanism in Nepal: *sarkar lai mat-labai chhaina* (government does not care about it). To get more benefit you should buy cheaper items from the Tarai and India and sell them here. How could you get good qualities of food at cheaper prices? Previously we had very few *rogs* (diseases) because we were eating homegrown food. Nowadays we go to the bazaar and buy a mixed or duplicate thing. I am not sure whether these types of food give you *tagat* (strength). Now the population has increased and we have to eat food from the bazaar and that is why we have many *rogs*. For example, if you eat the same variety of rice from your own field and rice from the market, you can get different a taste of it. The more you eat your homegrown food, the less you have to buy medicine and vitamin tonic from the market.

An additional perception is that *tagatilo* (nutritious) food can help to develop good health or to recover from conditions involving *dublo* (skinny) or *kamjor* (weakness). *Tagatilo* food are said to give strength, and make one *moto* (fat). Fatness is equated with good health, and to be called *moto* is highly complementary, especially for small children. *Dublo* (skinny) is associated with a weak and vulnerable state. This suggests the connection that to be *moto* is to be fed regularly a nutritious food. A thin person is considered unattractive as well as vulnerable to illness.

The notion of certain types of food as either strengthening or weakening the body is common in Kirtipur. I asked an elderly Newari woman to describe some representative food:

> Tea, coffee, tobacco and excess use of *rakshi* (alcohol) makes you weak. Strengthening types of food include green vegetables like mustard leaf, and other green leafy vegetables (*rayo, chumchur, pallungo*), so they are healthy. Other strengthening types of food are meat, fish, butter, lentil, potatoes and fresh fruits like apples, oranges, and bananas. Meat is very good, but it is not always affordable, that's why green vegetables and lentils are good. Strengthening types of food should be eaten daily, if you can afford them. Otherwise they should be eaten once a week. A new mother and growing children should specially eat these types of food. If there is a baby, the mother should eat, and the baby will get the food through the mother's milk.

Another woman emphasized the importance of *tagatilo* food when someone is taking medicine from allopathic doctors because: "If you are taking tablets or injections, it makes you weaker. Injection makes one weaker than tablets. In this case, you have to take *tagatilo* food like milk and fruits."

These examples show that the diet is perceived as an alternative to medicine in managing illness. Several respondents thought *tagatilo* food affected their behavior. For example, a young informant told me that he was reluctant to take allopathic medicine because: "unfortunately, I started to take allopathic medicine since my childhood because of my health problem. Whenever I have minor problems, I have to take high doses of medicine and it makes me weaker, and I need vitamin tonic."

Food as medicine and medicine as food

The hot–cold system usually overlaps with parallel food classification. Some examples have been quoted in the previous sections, such as "eat cold food for hot illnesses and hot food for cold illnesses." In the case of special physiological states such as pregnancy, lactation, and menstruation, certain types of food are sometimes avoided, or else prescribed to aid in the physiological process. Many women in Kirtipur, for example, told me that during lactation, taking *Jwano* soup could increase the supply of breast milk. Similarly, people with high blood pressure problems take lemon juice and sour oranges and avoid salty food, while the treatment of low blood pressure is supplemented by consuming salty food and red meat.

Many informants told me that if a person has a problem of *pathari* (gallstone or kidney stone) he/she should eat the soup of *gahat*. It is believed that the soup of *gahat* can split the stone into small pieces that leave the body through urination. Likewise, many medicines are regularly taken during meals as a symbolic form of food (Helman 1996).

Man, nature, and food

Moving to a different environment, to other *hawa-pani*, which literally means air and water, is also risky with regard to health. People's constitution is adjusted to the places where they live, and when moving from their natural environment, they are likely to fall ill. "This place is not suitable for me," is a typical expression. Moving to a different geographic place is seen as a health risk, as people in Nepal believe their constitution is suited to their place of origin. People from the hills are skeptical towards living in the lowlands, and people from the lowlands believe they will become sick in the hills.

The phrase *joro aayo* ("I got fever") was common in Kirtipur. I gave the person a scheme for classifying illnesses that the patients perceived as a result of a change in the body temperature – either hot or cold. In general, these feelings of abnormal temperature changes are purely subjective and bear little or no relation to a biomedical definition of normal body temperature as 98.4°F, (37°C). The conditions in which the patient feels hot are classified as *joro* (fever), those where he/she feels cold are classified as *thandi lagyo* or *chiso lagyo* (getting cold). Both fevers and colds are perceived as disequilibrium, which in the lay explanatory model have different causes, different effects, and thus require different treatments.

A combination of heat and cold seems to be manifested in the disease, not in the food. Thus, heat from the environment, bodily heat, and heat from food, all combine to produce hot diseases, and environmental cold, constitutional cold, and cold from food combine to produce cold diseases. A disease is a direct threat to life and cause of much anxiety, which needs to be explained and rationalized. Indeed, the system of hot–cold beliefs appears to be primarily an attempt to explain diseases and the classification of food seems secondary to this.

Night air, whether warm or cold, is considered dangerous, especially for children. A woman said: "Children get sick if you leave the bedroom window open at night." The skin protects the body from cold, but some areas are more vulnerable, such as the top of the head, the back of the neck, and the feet are exposed to both hot and cold conditions. For example, getting one's feet wet, walking around with bare feet, going out into the rain without an umbrella, could cause cold. Clothes prevent these body parts to be exposed to excessive hot or cold conditions.

A cold is caused by carelessness, stupidity, or lack of foresightedness. As an informant put it: "You get a cold when you don't dress properly. You go outside without enough clothes, wash your hair when you don't feel well and take excessive amount of cold foods during the cold seasons . . . and so on." Exposing oneself to cold types of food or a cold environment can cause one to catch cold (*sardi lagyo* or *thandi lagyo* or *chiso pasyo*). If, despite adequate precautions, one still gets a cold, it penetrates the boundaries of the human organism. According to Jitananda Joshi, a tantric-cum-Ayurvedic healer in Kirtipur, cold moves from the head down to the nose (causing a runny nose), the *pinas* (sinusitis, a head cold), and the chest (slight causing slight cough). It can travel even further downwards to the abdomen to cause vague abdominal discomfort and possibly slight inability to move, or to frequent bladder discomfort, but no burning sensation or fever. From damp feet it can migrate upwards to cause a stomach cold or cold to the bladder, or even further upwards to the nose, chest, or sinuses. All of these symptoms are accompanied by a subjective feeling of cold, shivering, and possibly by some muscular discomfort.

In the battle with environmental cold, one should strengthen one's own defense by dressing warmly, avoiding cold places, and building up the body's strength from within, by good food and potent tonics. If you did not eat properly, you were more liable to develop a cold. Treatment aims primarily to fight cold with warmth, and to move the patient from cold (or colder than normal) back to normal, by adding heat in the form of food and drinks, hot-water bottles, rest in the warm bed, and the like.

Food for gods, goddesses, and hungry ghosts

Gods and goddesses, locally called *bhagwan* or *devi-devata*, were most frequently worshiped in Kirtipur so that the devotee would obtain *punya* (merit). People believed that devotion establishes a social relation that is based on a hierarchical exchange where the gods and men are committed to each other. This may be in the hope of good fortune in this life and good faith after death. These gods demand and accept differing kinds of offerings. People believed that the gods protect the village by, for instance, patrolling the village boundary or guarding designated parts of the village. They also protect various social segments, families, and lineages in the village.

People also fed the gods, the goddesses, and the evil spirits for prevention and treatment of illnesses. First, the higher deities in general received raw food, whereas, the *lagu* (spirits which can attack a person) received cooked food. Second, devotees generally offered deities what they themselves were permitted to eat by the *jat* position. Even Brahmins might offer chicken and eggs to evil spirits, as long as the *Janne Manchhe* has prescribed it. To offer food was, therefore, a technique to please and influence one another. An ill person tries to make gods, goddesses, and spirits happy by offering food. The very existence of many of the harmful supernatural forces rested on the idea of an interdependency among men that persists after death. Hungry ghosts or evil spirits (e.g. *bhut, pret, pisachs,* and *masan*) are in death manipulating the living. For their own survival (i.e. for food) they are making claims on their victims. The victims, on the other hand, offer food to the ghosts and seek different types of healers if the problem becomes complicated.

Concluding remarks

In order to judge whether a diet is adequate or not, it is not sufficient to know about various kinds of food grown or collected. The association between food systems and nutritional status is complex because it also depends on how people choose to use the food they have as well as on the quantity, seasonal availability, affordability, and quality of the food. Within a single community there may be times of scarcity during one or several years, differences in wealth and consumption between the households, access to land and food, and permission to eat according to sex, age, and status.

Every society has customs regarding what to eat and how to prepare the food. The rules about food prohibitions and taboos may control access to some kinds of food. Justification for these rules leads in a beneficial, harmless, or dangerous direction. There are beliefs and practices that are harmful for pregnant, postpartum, and lactating women, and for children under five. My argument is that hot–cold beliefs adversely affect small children and postpartum mothers during their first three weeks. A number of available types of food could serve to broaden and improve the child's diet, but prohibitive local rules stops people from doing so at a time when a small child is also likely to be exposed to different diseases. The child's nutritional needs for growth suffers due to the perceived risk of the child getting ill. Slow weight increase sometimes causes severe malnutrition, which, in turn, weakens the young child's ability to resist infections and to cope with, and recover from, infectious diseases.

Similarly, the mothers must be kept warm, and be fed only hot food. Green vegetables, pumpkins, cauliflower, cabbage, all easily available in Kirtipur, were considered to be cooling, but were largely prohibited to eat by the mothers. Similarly, easily accessible fruits like banana and orange were also prohibited. According to biomedical practitioners and nutritionist, these are vitamin-rich types of food that are thought to be beneficial, and should be eaten more during postnatal periods.

In a clinical sense, most humoral practices could fall in the harmless category. The support they provide seems important in people's everyday life as well as in preventive medicine. On the other hand, the threats to health are found in the dietary prohibitions associated with pregnancy, postpartum and lactation periods, and with illness. This chapter has illustrated that different types of food, and the attitudes, beliefs, and practices surrounding them, are closely related to the community's complex cultural pattern.

Note

1 A version of this chapter originally appeared as 'Explanatory Models of Food, Health and Illness Ideology in Newar Town of Kirtipur', in R. P. Chaudhary, B. Subedi, T. Aase and O. Vetas (eds.), *Vegetation and Society*, pp. 228–239 (Kathmandu: Tribhuvan University, Kathmandu and University of Bergen, Norway, 2002). Used with permission.

References

Blustain, H. S. 1976. "Levels of Medicine in a Central Nepali Village." *Contributions to Nepalese Studies* 3: 85–105.

Caplan, P. 1997. "Social and Cultural Implications of Food and Food Habits." In P. Caplan, ed., *Food, Health and Identity*. London: Routledge.

Cassel, J. 1977. "Social and Cultural Implication of Food and Food Habits." In David Landy, ed., *Culture, Disease and Healing: Studies in Medical Anthropology*, pp. 236–241. New York: Macmillan Publishing Co., Inc.

Chowdhury, A. Mumin, Cecil Helman and Trisha Greenhalgh. 2000. "Food Beliefs and Practice among British Bangladeshis with Diabetes: Implication for Health Education." *Anthropology & Medicine* 7(2): 209–226.

Foster, G. M. 1994. *Hippocrates' Latin American Legacy: Humoral Medicine in the New World.* New York: Gordon and Breach Science Publishers.

Geertz, C. 1973. *The Interpretation of Culture.* New York: Basic Books.

Good, B. J. 1994. *Medicine, Rationality and Experience: An Anthropological Perspective.* Cambridge: Cambridge University Press.

Helman, C. G. 1996. *Culture, Health and Illness: An Introduction for Health Professionals* (3rd Edition). Oxford: Butterworth-Heinemann.

Kleinman, A. 1978. "Concepts and Model for the Comparison of Medical Systems as Cultural Systems." *Social Science and Medicine* 12: 85–93.

Kleinman, A. 1980. *Patients and Healers in the Contexts of Culture.* Berkeley: University of California Press.

Lowdin, P. 1985. *Food Ritual and Society among the Newars.* Uppsala: Uppsala University, Department of Cultural Anthropology.

McElroy, A. and P. K. Townsend. 1996. *Medical Anthropology in Ecological Perspective* (3rd Edition). Colorado: Westview Press.

Pool, R. 1987. "Hot and Cold as an Explanatory Model: The Example of Bharuch District in Gujarat, India." *Social Science and Medicine* 25(4): 389–399.

Stone, L. 1976. "Concept of Illness and Curing in a Central Nepal Village." *Contributions to Nepalese Studies* 3: 55–80.

Subedi, M. S. 2001. *Medical Anthropology of Nepal.* Kathmandu: Udaya Books (P) Ltd.

6 Uterine prolapse

A mobile camp approach and body politics in Nepal[1]

Although the women's health agenda has been largely defined by biomedicine and public health, anthropology has much to offer in terms of defining and understanding women's health from the perspective of women themselves (Inhorn 2006). And the health problems, be it among men or women, cannot be separated from the larger social, cultural, economic, and political forces that shape and constrain human life. This chapter examines the prolapsed uterus, one of the major reproductive health problems of women in Nepal, and the short-term camp approach, perceptions of uterine prolapse (UP), and of different body parts in the local context. I also try to offer some policy issues for sustainable public health intervention.

UP is a condition in which a woman's supportive pelvic muscles, tissues, and ligaments break away from the body's internal structure and the uterus, rectum, or bladder drop into or out of the vagina. The condition is mainly due to insufficiency of the pelvic floor and consists of herniation of an adjacent pelvic organ into the vagina. UP is usually classified into three anatomical stages, corresponding to the severity of the condition. In the first stage, the uterus leaves its place but is still inside the vagina. In the second stage, the uterus leaves its place and moves to the opening of the vagina. For these two stages, conservative management including pelvic floor muscle training or ring pessary insertion are considered the best options (UNFPA and Sancharika Samuha 2007). A pessary is a plastic or rubber device that is inserted into the vagina, which holds the uterus. After a health worker inserts this into the vagina, there is no need to do anything for three months. Every three months, it has to be taken out, cleaned properly and inserted back after boiling in hot water. If a woman becomes pregnant while the pessary is inserted, it must be taken out in a health institution. The pessary cannot hold the uterus in a situation where the uterus is fully out.

In the third stage, the uterus comes out of the vagina, and the woman must go to a hospital to be treated through surgical procedures by trained doctors. Mostly these surgeries involve surgical removal of the uterus and subsequently a pelvic floor repair. After the surgery, the women will be able to perform their normal work, but will not be able to undergo menstruation or become pregnant.

For the most part, Nepal adheres to traditional gender roles where women are not always able to make independent decisions about their reproductive health. But families and communities still refuse to speak about the disease and it is often a secret kept within the home (UNFPA and Sancharika Samuha 2007). The causes and consequences of the problem as perceived by women suffering from UP, government initiative to address this issue, and socio-cultural practices regarding UP, will be discussed in the following sections.

Methods and materials

The research was done by the author while participating in mobile camps operated by Adventist Development and Relief Agency (ADRA) Nepal in the Jumla, Bajura, and Achham districts, and by Public Health Concern Trust (PHECT) Nepal in the Salyan district. Although the objective of the field visit was to conduct a final evaluation of the mobile health camp projects implemented by ADRA and PHECT-Nepal, the author, being an anthropologist, collected additional information regarding socio-cultural issues of UP and the ethnography of the mobile camps. These issues are pertinent but were beyond the scope of the project evaluation itself.

Interaction with the women suffering from UP was done in detail to find out the social and cultural practices regarding reproductive and sexual health issues. Such interactions were conducted in an exploratory fashion, mainly by generally asking about the health situation in their locality and subsequently shifting to the women's general health problems. Slowly the interaction concentrated on the illness the women generally suffer from. The informants were further probed to discuss UP issues. Focus group discussions (FGD) with women and men and interactions with the mobile health camp team and local health workers at the concerned health facilities were also conducted to validate the information and get more insight regarding UP related issues. Men were included in the study in order to achieve community perspectives. Moreover, a series of interactions were done with the women who were waiting for surgery and who had undergone surgical correction at the Nepalganj Medical College Teaching Hospital,

Kohalpur. Though there are issues related to quality of care and of the management at the campsites and the hospital, the chapter is limited to causes, consequences, and cultural perceptions regarding UP. This does not mean that quality of care and process management issues are less important. This, however, belongs to another article.

Results and discussion

Prevalence of prolapsed uterus

The global prevalence of prolapsed uterus ranges from 4 percent to 40 percent (UK APPG 2009, cited in Pradhan et al. 2010). Studies in Nepal have shown varying prevalence for Nepal. A study conducted by (Bonetti et al. 2004) in Far-Western Nepal revealed that 25 percent of the visitors to free female health care clinics were diagnosed with UP. In their study in Bhaktapur, Marahatta and Shah (2003) found that prevalence of UP among women aged 20 years and above was 8 percent. Another study (Tuladhar 2005) conducted in the Bajhang district found that 51.6 percent of the visitors to a medical camp for women had gynecological problems, of which 36 percent were UP.

The 2006 Nepal Demographic and Health Survey (NDHS) found that up to 7 percent of women of reproductive age (15–49 years) suffered from UP (MoHP, New ERA, and Macro International Inc. 2007) The 2011 NDHS also reported that 6 percent of women who had ever given birth had experienced symptoms of uterine prolapse. Among these women 55 percent sought medical treatment, 9 percent sought traditional treatment, and 36 percent did not seek any treatment at all (MoHP, New ERA, and ICF International Inc. 2012).

A study of reproductive morbidity done by The Institute of Medicine and UNFPA (2006) among a representative sample of 2,070 women in 8 districts in rural and urban areas in the 163 hills and in Tarai, showed a 10.4 percent prevalence of UP. This study estimated that 600,000 women in Nepal suffer from UP, the majority of these women were of reproductive age, and about 200,000 women were eligible for curative surgery (Institute of Medicine and UNFPA 2006). Among them, 25.2 percent were below the age of 35, including 2.8 percent in the adolescent age group (15–19 years). Women above 30 years were the most vulnerable, 45.1 percent among them having UP. Among women 20 years and below, 14 percent had UP for the first time. Among 30.4 percent of the women, UP was first noted after the first delivery, 44.9 percent noted after the second and third deliveries. The mean number of years of suffering from UP problems was 7.89 years. Among them, 4.3 percent had suffered for 21–30 years.

Unlike in the developed world where UP is commonly seen in the postmenopausal age group unrelated to child birth, UP in Nepal was registered among a younger population. The mean age for the first occurrence of prolapsed uterus was 27.91 years, which indicates that women suffer UP for many years, beginning at a relatively young age. Unlike our firm belief that UP is more common in the hilly regions, this study showed that the prevalence of UP was higher in the Tarai districts in southern Nepal. Among the women diagnosed with reproductive health problems, 44.5 percent and 27.6 had UP problems in Rautahat and Saptari, respectively. In Dadeldhura, the prevalence of UP was 17.7 percent. Thus, the study clearly showed that UP was a serious public health problem in all of Nepal's ecological zones and development regions (Institute of Medicine and UNFPA 2006). High prevalence of UP is a symptom of a larger problem concerning reproductive rights and access to education and information.

Causes of UP

Marriage is assumed to be a basic, vital, and fundamental institution not only for the physical, mental, spiritual, and social comfort of the spouses, but for the maintenance, protection, and education of the progeny. After marriage, the wife lives in the husband's home, and she has to consider the husband's family also as her family. She must, therefore, adjust herself to the changed situation after her marriage. She has to look upon her mother-in-law and father-in-law as her own mother and father. Thus, the marriage is a sacramental process whereby the woman is transferred as a gift from one household to another. Motherhood is one of the carvings of a normal woman – no authority needs to be cited to support this view (Uberoi 1996). Parties enter into marriage alliances on the assumption that they will become a father and a mother in the due course of time (Subedi 2001). Having children is one of the principal aims of marriage, it is assumed that women have an innate desire for motherhood, which in the proper course should be satisfied, that men too have a deep, although more culturally grounded, desire for parenthood, and that the joint procreation of children cements and reinforces the conjugal bond. It is a more common experience that the birth of a child, preferably a son, puts an end to minor misunderstandings and bickering between the spouses, for the partners to concentrate on lavishing in a common love of the child and thus being brought together. Contrariwise, a wife who is not prepared to become a mother at the cost of her youth, or who aborts a fetus against her husband's wishes, is imputed to be unnatural, irresponsible, and cruel.

In Nepal, the level of awareness regarding the need to rest before and after child birth is very low. The mother-in-law, generally, shares the events during the delivery days of the babies. They generally feel that birth is normal and there is no need for special arrangement before, during, and after the delivery. Such attitude hinders an awareness of the need for, and the importance of, institutional delivery, the importance of rest after delivery, and to minimize physical work immediately after the delivery. Furthermore, such situations within the family discourage pregnant women to take measures that can prevent UP.

During the mobile camps, many women shared with us stories such as,

> many mother-in-laws still tell their daughter-in-laws that their own first birth was given in the jungle when they were collecting grass and firewood for household use. The second birth was given when planting rice or millet in the field, and the third birth was given when they were in the market to buy household goods.

The ultimate message shared is that there is no need to rest before and during delivery. They further mentioned that young family members have been more aware about the importance of antenatal care and institutional delivery. However, due to household work, the practices of collecting firewood from the forest, water to be collected from long distances due to unavailability of tap water in or near the household, and due to lack of supportive family members, many women are forced to work immediately after delivery.

Women in Nepal carry heavy loads after child birth, work strenuously, and cannot maintain a nutritious diet. Research (Bonetti et al. 2004; Bodner-Adler et al. 2007; Dangal 2008) and gynecologists have identified several causes for UP: a large number of child births or spacing successive child births too close to each other; giving birth at a tender age; lack of nutritious food during pregnancy and after child birth; unsafe miscarriages and abortions; pressure to the lower abdomen before the delivery stage as well as after child birth; the weakening of the pelvic floor where the uterus rests; the pelvis separating from the pelvic floor while giving birth; insufficient child birth tools; giving birth to a large baby through the vagina; attempts to give birth by pressing the stomach for a long time during the delivery period; continuously coughing after child birth; applying more pressure than required before the time of child birth; lifting heavy objects after child birth; malnutrition; dysentery for a long period; lack of blood; and lack of rest after child birth. Many of these conditions are common in rural Nepal.

Women's memories of first events of uterine prolapse

Almost all women in this study were reluctant to share their first memories of UP events, probably, I assume, because they had problems with sharing such experiences in front of a male. After informal discussions about the causes of UP, and also telling them about similar problems in other districts, they became more open and started to share their memories. They were, however, also concerned about their identity in the stories that would be written about them. After being assured that their privacy would be strictly maintained, they shared their first memories openly.

> After 7 days of the birth of my child, I had to cook food, fetch water and take care of cows and buffalos. My uterine could not tighten after giving birth. One day when I was carrying water in a *gagri* (copper vessel) from the public tap, my uterine muscles loosened, causing the womb to fall slightly. With each successive pregnancy and continuous heavy work – farming, fetching water, collecting firewood and fodder – the problem got worse. After my sixth delivery, the whole uterus came out.

These are the words of a 42-year-old woman in Salyan. She continued: "I was too shy and did not tell anybody. I used to push it back into my body." A woman aged 35 in Bajura said: "After two weeks of my second delivery, I had gone to the forest to collect *daura* (firewood) for cooking food. After returning from the forest with the heavy load of firewood, I suddenly felt that my uterus was falling down with pain."

The story of another woman from Achham is not that much different. A woman of 45 told us:

> When I was 16, I gave the first birth, but the child survived only 15 days. Next year I gave the second birth. The baby survived only one year. The third delivery was a son who is now 25 years old. After my fourth delivery, I felt weak. I was very thin. One day, I was climbing the tree to collect the fodder and I felt uneasy. I was sweating. Later it fell.

A 32-year-old woman in Salyan said: "I had just given birth to my first child and was working in the fields near my village. Suddenly I felt as if my insides were dropping out of me. I told no one – not even my husband – hoping the problem would go away." Many women shared similar stories. A feeling of heaviness in the lower abdomen and pain in the lower abdomen were other memories of UP. Due to fear, they could not share their problems even with their husbands.

Consequences of uterus prolapse

The women were hesitant to discuss their problems with UP, due to shame and humiliation. Many women fear condemnation from their communities and families, and the disease is not openly discussed and debated within the family and in society. Women who suffer from UP continue to be silent on the matter.

Many women shared with us that they faced urinating difficulties, *tallo pet duckhne* (lower abdominal pain), *seto ganaune pani bagne* (foul smelling white discharge). Other difficulties mentioned were lifting, standing, walking, and painful intercourse. Women suffering from a second- or third-degree uterine prolapse were unable to walk or stand. A 49-year-old woman in Jumla told us: "I did not have enough food. I didn't go to the doctor. My uterus kept falling out and I suffered a lot. I could not move, and I was in pain while working. My husband started to beat me and threatened to take a second wife. My mother-in-law thought I was not working well enough." She continued: "The health post was a 2 hour walking distance from my house. I had visited it previously for stomach pain and a wound. It was difficult for me to walk, and had abdominal pain due to UP, but I did not discuss the curability of my misery of a prolapsed uterus." Feeling ashamed to share their reproductive health problems with the health workers was very common. Some women mentioned that they had a relatively good relationship with their husband. They blamed their fate.

This debilitating condition exposed the women to rejection by their husbands, family, and sometimes even by the community. As a result, they are completely deprived of their rights to participate in the society, including in the community's development activities. Responding to the consequences of UP, the reproductive health expert from UNFPA who had been coordinating the mobile camp said: "The consequence of UP is very pathetic. It is cheaper for a man to leave his wife and marry again. I have heard such stories in far-western mountain districts. Insulting women because of prolapse is very common." These examples provide enough documentation for the urgent need to study UP-related social stigma and develop appropriate health education and promotion materials to prevent UP.

Almost all the interviewed women were unaware that treatment was available. A woman who had undergone surgical correction told us that they would routinely push the uterus back in place, to have it drop out again when coughing or sneezing. In Achham, I also noticed that the women with UP problems were called *Dhauki*, a term used to dehumanize women suffering from UP. Research findings conducted in Nepal show that such deprivation has great consequences (Bonetti et al. 2004).

The camp approach: experimentation and learning

The Government of Nepal has recognized uterine prolapse as a high priority condition and has shown its commitment by creating a fund for providing free uterine prolapse surgery services to women in need. In September 2007, Director of Family Health Division, Department of Health Services stated that in 2006 the government provided funds for free treatment of about 3,000–5,000 women. The camp approach has been used in family planning and for cataract operation for many years in Nepal. Since 2005, reproductive health services (including family planning, emergency obstetric care, and treatment for prolapsed uterus) have been delivered in remote areas through mobile reproductive health camps. To support this effort, reproductive health mobile camps have been organized periodically with support from the UNFPA and donors like the European Union and the Danish, British, and Japanese governments.

The camp approach means that additional services related to reproductive health are provided to the marginalized, underserved, and conflict affected people in Nepal. The long-term plan is to improve the reproductive health, protection, and self-sufficiency status of the most vulnerable parts of the population. The immediate objectives of the camps are to increase reproductive as well as general health services; to ensure delivery of essential reproductive health services through mobile outreach health camps to women, men, and adolescents; and to strengthen delivery of reproductive health services through the primary health care approach ensuring essential medical supplies and relevant kits. The camp approach includes information, education, and communication activities to generate the demand and provision of high quality services closer to the community.

Observations from some mobile health camps

The camps take place on a special day, with the help of experts coming from higher levels within or outside the formal health system. During the camps, patients are screened for UP and severe cases are sent to the hospital where a team of specialists conducts the operations. The surgery and medication are free of charge and each patient, with one attendant, is provided travel and food expenses. These services are likely to be expanded in the future. However, a clear vision and strategy has not been adapted to shift from humanitarian aid to a more sustainable public health intervention owned by the government.

The date and place for the camps are, generally, decided by the consensus of the district-based stakeholders, and this information is distributed to the people in the respective districts from different sources, ranging from Female Community Health Workers (FCHV), youth clubs, mother's groups, pamphlets, posters, and from the local FM radio stations. On the camp day, various camp management activities are conducted in a very systematic way. Near the entrance gate is the registration counter where the health workers fill out a specially designed camp sheet for registering basic socio-demographic information for each case. Volunteers guide each patient to the appropriate room for history taking.

The second counter is for history taking and general examination. The local health facility staff or junior health staff takes a detailed history about the person and fill it in the form. The history includes obstetric, menstrual history, and major complaints. The doctor or the nurse also examines weight, pulse, blood pressure, and checks for anemia or jaundice. The health worker tells the clients about internal examination and also motivates them for undergoing vaginal and abdominal examination. If the client refuses, then the treatment is given on the basis of the symptoms only. If the client agrees, she is sent for a detailed examination by a doctor.

The third station is for internal examination in a separate room with provisions made for privacy. The doctor carries out the vaginal and abdominal examination after reviewing the history of the client. Common problems such as reproductive tract infection, prolapse, etc., if found, are demonstrated by the medical doctor to the nurses or the health staff working at the local health facility as part of their training. The doctor prescribes the medicine and briefly explains the management to the clients. If required, the client is referred to the laboratory for simple tests such as hemoglobin and urine tests. After doing the lab test the client returns to the specialist for further consultation and treatment.

The next station is for counseling and guidance to explain the patient the details of her problems and how to take medicines and further preventive measures. This is done by the health educator, a public health nurse, or a reproductive health counselor. Cases who need further treatment at a higher level such as a prolapse operation are referred to the appropriate level of services by giving them a written referral slip. Finally the clients go to the dispensing counter to collect the medicines prescribed. The camps provide free medicine especially for women's reproductive health problems.

An exhibition is also set up for providing health education on various aspects. The clients can see the exhibition while they are waiting to be examined by the specialists. The clients' relatives can also see the exhibition while they are waiting. The information, education, and communication (IEC) activities include posters and pamphlets, interaction and a targeted media campaign, video show, and street drama. The influences of social, cultural, and economic conditions on health are taken into consideration in the IEC activities. Identifying and promoting specific types of behavior that are desirable are usually the objectives of the IEC efforts.

Every staff member is given specific duties during the camp. For example, the Auxiliary Nurse Midwife (ANM) and nurses take the history and assist during the internal examination. Local volunteers help with the registration, weighing, provide health education, and assist with general arrangements. The health educator provides health education to women who are waiting. The clients' attendance at the camp depends on the season, agricultural work, and also publicity.

The camp ends with a review meeting where the problems related to the organization of the camp, the type of cases seen and the follow-up required, any difficulties faced and lessons learned are discussed among the team members. Some implementing partners arrange meetings to share experiences with the local health facility staff and the community people separately to listen to their impressions from the camp activities.

The uterine prolapse cases requiring surgical correction are referred to tertiary care centers. Most of them are managed by Nepalganj Medical College Teaching Hospital. It has become a referral hub for surgical correction for uterine prolapse cases for almost all funded projects in the Mid-Western and Far-Western regions. However, no mechanism is developed for post-discharge consultation or responsibility for the patients who underwent surgical corrections. After the surgical correction and due stay at a hospital, some women faced difficulties while returning home because they had to travel long distances from Nepalganj to their respective districts. Some of the patients mentioned having complications such as pain and infections in the operated areas, and had to consult and make purchases at local pharmacists.

When inquiring at the local health facilities about the women who were referred for surgery and about complications faced after surgery, we found that the information regarding such issues were not provided by the implementing partners. People from the District Health Office (DHO) had visited the mobile camps, but they were just informal visits. A clear-cut monitoring and information system to keep track of these patients who have undergone surgical procedures, especially the ones who could face complications, seem to be absent.

Many people responded positively to the camps in all the places that I visited during this study. "The camp approach has provided an opportunity for women to break their 'culture of silence' about various reproductive health problems. Women have started to share such problems with their neighbors, relatives, and health facility staff," said a local teacher in Jumla. Another teacher mentioned that the camp approach was like a "buffet party in a good hotel" or "catering services during feasts," and that a variety of technical experts including health educators were available. People also got a chance to watch reproductive health related documentaries, participate in organized dramas, and eat, and talk with outsiders. Once the camps are over, nothing will remain, and people have to survive as usual.

On the other hand, a female community health worker in Salyan who was working for the camp management said:

> The camp approach has encouraged many women to share their health problems with the doctors. Women in the community go to be examined on the camp day where they get support from each other. Such camps where women are properly examined with due privacy and care help to change the norm in the community where unnecessary modesty prevents early diagnosis of many reproductive illnesses and proper management of such problems.

However, during a focus group discussion with males in Jumla, some respondents had a slightly different opinion regarding mobile camps. They compared camps with catering services and buffet party during picnic, wedding ceremonies, and feasts. They said that one can see and get all kinds of services for three days and nothing would remain after the camps. Their concern was to address the basic needs, promote sustainable health, and strengthen the districts' existing health facilities.

A 44-year-old woman from Bajura, who had undergone surgery six months earlier in Nepalganj Medical College Teaching Hospital told us:

> I had been suffering from white discharges and lower abdominal pain for 15 years, a long time. I was very shy to discuss this with

anyone until I heard them broadcast on the radio about the free health camps. Even though I was initially reluctant to share my problems with the person at the registration (since he was a male), I gathered enough courage to tell him my problem. The female doctor was open, polite and assuring, and listened to all my problems patiently and prescribed me the medication along with clear instructions about how and when to use them. And here I am today, all healthy and happy with no such problems whatsoever.

In this approach special resources are mobilized periodically for a short time rather than providing high level services continuously in rural areas. In a camp or campaign, I found that the health staff at a local health facility was active and willing to put extra efforts and work as a team. Services given at a higher level also attracted the community as they see more value in less time and effort. However, there was not a long-term perspective of service at the community level.

Learning experiences from the camp approach are that because it is a very short-term activity, the issue of sustainability is questionable. Camps should be run on a more routine and regular basis, and also be smaller so that better quality of services can be ensured. The community should also know in advance that the camp activity will take place on a fixed day of the month. This would enable people to plan to go to the camp, the number of clients would probably be lower, thus giving more time for individual attention to the clients. The cost of the camps will also be reduced because many of the services become routine with little outside input.

Medicine like vaginal tablets and higher antibiotics were given to the women from the camp pharmacy. Such medicines were not available in the permanent local health facilities, and were not included as essential medicine. During the interaction with the women, they told us that they later bought the same medicine with the help of the prescription provided during the mobile camps, often with the help of their relatives and friends who had gone to the district headquarters or to Nepalganj. The women did this because the medicines were effective, but were not available at the local health facility. Thus, the camp approach has accelerated the use of medicine in the remote areas.

Body politics: barriers to accessing care

Until recently, social and political theory and scholarship tended to ignore the human body, placing emphasis upon social structure and individual subjectivity with little discussion of where the 'lived body' fitted in (Lupton 2003). One reason for the reluctance to theorize or historically position the body was, in my view, the desire of scholars in the humanities and the social sciences to avoid the biological determinism of the hard human sciences. As a result, for decades, macro-sociologists have tended to focus on the social system, the structural, political, and economic dimensions of social control, a theoretical space in which the body was absent, while micro-sociologists were concerned with individual behavior as socially constituted, but neglected considerations of the embodiment of the decision making. How individuals can regulate themselves and control their bodily deportment was the central concern of this study.

Foucault (1979) identified the establishment of medical clinics and teaching hospitals in the late 18th century as a pivotal point for conceptualizing the body. In *The Birth of the Clinic* (1975), Foucault described changes in medical practices during the 18th century: the introduction and routine adoption of physical examination; the postmortem; the stethoscope; the microscope; the development of the discipline of anatomy, psychiatry, radiology, and surgery; and the institutionalization of the hospital and the doctor's surgery, all of which served to increasingly exert power upon the body. At the same time, bodies were subjected to increased regulation, constant monitoring, discipline, and surveillance in other spheres, most notably in prisons, in schools, in asylums, in the military, and in professional workshops. The medical encounter began to demand that patients reveal the secrets of their bodies, both by allowing physical examination and by giving their medical history when questioned by doctors. The patients had to speak, to confess, to reveal; illness was transformed from what is visible to what was heard.

For Foucault, the medical encounter was a supreme example of surveillance, whereby the doctor investigates, questions, touches the patient's exposed flesh, while the patient acquiesces and confesses, with little knowledge of why the procedures are carried out. The body is rendered an object to be prodded, tested, and examined. The owner is expected to give up to the doctor his/her jurisdiction of the body. The sexually active body is currently a primary site at which contesting discourses compete for meaning, particularly in the field of medicine and public health (Lupton 2003).

Most people in Nepal are socialized at a very early age into society's norms concerning the situations, circumstances, and purposes of allowable and unallowable genital exposure. Females in particular are socialized into rigorous norms concerning society's expectations to cover specific private areas of her body, especially the genital parts. Even for a woman who has overcome being bothered by genital exposure in the presence of her sexual partner, this problem frequently recurs when she is expected to expose her vagina in a nonsexual manner to a male medical doctor.

This is the case with vaginal examination (Henslin and Biggs 1991) during a reproductive health check-up. In fact, vaginal examination can become so threatening that for many women it not only represents a threat to their feelings of modesty, but also threatens them as a person and their feelings of who they are. The reason is that through learning about taboos, emotions often are associated with the genital area, thus nudity and undressing in front of strangers are problematic for the patient. Clothing is considered as an extension of the self, and in some cases the clothing comes to represent the particular part of the body that it covers. In this case, this means that panties and girdles represent women's 'private area'. Conceptualizing the vagina as a sacred object yields a perspective that appears to be of value in analyzing vaginal examination. Sacred objects are surrounded by rules protecting the objects from being profaned, rules governing who may approach the sacred, under what circumstances it may be approached, and what may and may not be done during such an approach (Durkheim 1995). If these rules are followed, the sacred will not lose any of its sacredness, but if they are violated, there is a danger of the sacred being profaned.

By conceptualizing the vagina in this way, who may and who may not approach the vagina is highly circumscribed, with the primary person so allowed being one who is ritually related to the possessor of the vagina, the husband (Henslin and Biggs 1991). It is perhaps because they have profaned the sacred that prostitutes usually lack respect. And in doing so, not only have they failed to limit vaginal access to culturally prescribed individuals, they have added further violation by allowing vaginal access on a pecuniary basis. They have, in effect, sold the sacred (Henslin and Biggs 1991).

Uterine prolapse is a complex condition affecting a sensitive part of the woman's body. Therefore, it is associated with shame and often kept secret. Many women fear condemnation from their communities and families, and discussions and debates about the disease do not openly occur within the family and in society. Women who suffer from uterine prolapse continue to remain silent about the matter. A woman in Salyan having a second-degree prolapse said: "How could I tell others? It's such a shameful thing." A FCHV from the same health facility mentioned: "Many women in the village are living with such problems for more than 30–40 years. They cannot tell about their problems to the doctors, but just say they have pain in the lower abdomen and turn their heads down. If a doctor is not experienced, he/she would not be able to diagnose the real problem."

During the camp observations and in-depth interviews with the female community health workers in Achham, we found that it was difficult for these women to share uterine prolapse problems with the local health workers. The doctor at the camp told that a female community health worker suffering from UP problems could not share her problem directly with the doctor. When the doctor asked to examine her uterus, she did not give permission. After an hour's consulting and detailed checking of the body, she was diagnosed with a second-degree prolapsed uterus.

The results from the study by the Institute of Medicine and UNFPA (2006) revealed that 46.97 percent waited for 15–30 years before seeking treatment in a hospital. Such a long time before seeking treatment is due to deep-rooted socio-cultural aspects regarding UP. The women who know where they can be treated and have the means to go there, hesitate due to fear of divorce or abandonment, isolation, shame, and sensitivity surrounding genital issues, due to the traditional belief that hysterectomies will lead to weakness, and to a lack of emotional support.

Many women face obstacles in receiving necessary follow-up care, particularly regarding pessary rings, which requires periodic replacement by a medical practitioner and maintenance to avoid infection. Discussions with women with uterine prolapse in Salyan and Achham, and with the camp team, revealed that some women had been using the same ring for more than two years, and consequently developed an infection. They had inserted a pessary during the health camps or at the tertiary health care center, but were not aware of its proper management. They were hesitant to talk about it with the health workers at the local health facility, and the local health workers did not know that the particular women had inserted it.

Conclusion

Although uterine prolapse is not an immediately life-threatening condition, it seriously hampers the quality of life of those who are affected. For women living with this condition, life's basic activities are challenged. Urinating, defecating, walking, standing, sitting, and sexual intercourse can be difficult and painful. This, in turn, leads to various forms of psychological, social, and physical impairments. Surgical treatments of advanced stages of UP cannot be a substitute for preventive measures. Extensive information and preventive programs as well as early management of genital prolapse should be the first steps to reduce this significant social and public health problem in Nepal. A substantial shift from humanitarian aid to more sustainable public health interventions, and strengthening the existing health facilities in the districts and regions, is urgent. Similarly, there is a need to assess the health related quality of life that can be gained through uterine prolapse surgery. At the same time, interdisciplinary research, combining biomedical and social science methods, should be promoted so that epidemiological information as well as a clear understanding of the context in which health problems arise can be obtained.

Note

1 A version of this chapter originally appeared as 'Uterine Prolapse, Mobile Health Camp Approach and Body Politics in Nepal', *Dhaulagiri Journal of Sociology and Anthropology*, 4: 21–40, 2010. Used with permission.

References

Bodner-Adler, Barbara, Chanda Shrivastava and Klaus Bodner. 2007. "Risk Factors for Uterine Prolapse in Nepal." *International Urogynecology Journal* 18: 1343–1346.

Bonetti, Tiphaine, Anne Erpelding and Laxmi Raj Pathak. 2004. "Listening to 'Felt Needs': Investigating Genital Prolapse in Western Nepal." *Reproductive Health Matters* 12(23): 166–175.

Dangal, Ganesh. 2008. "A Study of Reproductive Morbidity of Women in Eastern Terai Region of Nepal." *Nepal Journal of Obstetrics and Gynecology* 3(1): 29–34.

Durkheim, Emile. 1995. *The Elementary Forms of Religious Life*. Translated by Karen Fields. New York: Free Press.

Foucault, M. 1975. *The Birth of the Clinic: An Archaeology of Medical Perception*. New York: Vintage Books.

Foucault, M. 1979. *The History of Sexuality, Volume One: An Introduction*. London: Penguin.

Henslin, James M. and Mae A. Biggs. 1991. "The Sociology of Vaginal Examination." In James M. Henslin, ed., *Down to Earth Sociology*. New York: The Free Press.

Inhorn, Marcia C. 2006. "Defining Women's Health: A Dozen Messages from More than 150 Ethnographies." *Medical Anthropology Quarterly* 20(3): 345–378.

Institute of Medicine and UNFPA. 2006. *Status of Reproductive Morbidities in Nepal*. Kathmandu: Report Submitted to UNFPA.

Lupton, Deborah. 2003. *Medicine as Culture*. London: Sage Publications.

Marahatta, R. K. and Arati Shah. 2003. "Genital Prolapse in Women of Bhaktapur." *Nepal Medical College Journal* 5(1): 31–33.

MoHP, New ERA, and ICF International Inc. 2012. *Nepal Demographic and Health Survey 2011*. Kathmandu: MoHP, New ERA, and Macro International Inc.

MoHP, New ERA, and Macro International Inc. 2007. *Nepal Demographic and Health Survey 2006*. Kathmandu: MoHP, New ERA, and Macro International Inc.

Pradhan, Ajit, Bal Krishna Subedi, Sarah Barnett, Sharad Kumar Sharma, Mahesh Puri, Pradeep Poudel, Sovana Raj Chitrakar, Naresh Pratap K. C. and Louise Hulton. 2010. *Nepal Maternal Mortality and Morbidity Study 2008/2009*. Kathmandu: Family Health Division, Ministry of Health and Population.

Subedi, Madhusudan. 2001. *Medical Anthropology of Nepal*. Kathmandu: Udaya Books.

Tuladhar, H. 2005. "An Overview of Reproductive Health of Women in Bajhang District." *Nepal Medical College Journal* 7(2): 107–111.

Uberoi, Patricia. 1996. "When Is a Marriage Not a Marriage? Sex, Sacrament and Contract in Hindu Marriage." *Contributions to Indian Sociology: Occasional Studies* 7: 319–345.

UNFPA and Sancharika Samuha. 2007. *Booklet on Uterine Prolapse*. Kathmandu: Sancharika Samuha.

7 Communication aspects in health care work in Nepal[1]

Madhusudan Subedi and Marit Bakke

Communication is about exchanging ideas, information, and knowledge. It is also about transferring new ideas, information, and knowledge from people who know to people who do not know. This is done in order to change people's ideas and to increase their knowledge about different issues, often with the intention of also changing people's behavior. Such communication processes are very important when we are interested in social development which can improve people's social and economic conditions. However, we must emphasize that although communication is an important tool for handling social problems, not all problems are communication problems. Why this is so will be discussed later in this chapter.

Good health is fundamentally and intrinsically important for living a worthwhile human life and for individuals to participate in the development of a society. This is the case throughout the world, but even more so in developing countries. For instance, former Director-General of the WHO, Gro Harlem Brundtland (1999: vii) stated that "Remarkable gains in health, rapid economic growth and unprecedented scientific advance – all legacies of the 20th century – could lead us to a new era of human progress." She continued (ibid.: viii):

> Opportunity entails responsibility. Working together we have the opportunity to transform lives now debilitated by disease and fear of economic ruin into lives filled with realistic hopes. I have pledged to place health at the core of the global development agenda. That is where it belongs. Wise investments in health can prove to be the most successful strategies to lead people out of poverty.

This is indeed an ambitious vision, particularly when we discuss how it can be implemented in different countries with specific economic, social, physical, and cultural conditions. It is often argued that good health services are crucial for improving people's health condition. Research has shown (e.g. Justice 1986; Dixit 1999; Subedi 2001) and health workers know from experience, that the presence of health services is not sufficient because many people do not use them due to physical/geographic, economic, and cultural barriers. The process of exclusion and the existence of cultural conditions join in an alliance that is very unfortunate for certain vulnerable groups. Also access to all other human development resources is a crucial prerequisite for enhancing people's living condition in general, and for improving their health in particular.

Any communication process or strategy must focus on a particular issue or message. In this chapter the issue is how communication can be used to cope with malnutrition and certain types of illnesses that are prevalent among the Nepalese population. The next section describes some facts about health conditions and health services in Nepal. Then follows a brief introduction to different development paradigms as well as an assessment of their relevance for social change. The next section describes some basic principles in communication theory, being explored further in the following section. This section includes a presentation of a communication strategy in which people get a chance to express cultural beliefs with respect to health and treatment practices, and how this knowledge can be applied to facilitate increased use of health services. To include indigenous health, knowledge must be considered seriously in such a strategy. Thus, the challenge is to find ways to apply people's beliefs and knowledge as a basis for establishing health services in which knowledge from indigenous health practices as well as from school medicine can be merged. The last section illustrates the importance of being aware of cultural preconditions by presenting terms used by mothers in five different ethnic groups in Nepal to describe acute respiratory infections (ARI) and illnesses among children, one of the country's major health problems.

Health conditions and health care in Nepal

Over the last 50 years, considerable gains in the health status have been achieved. There has been considerable progress in offering the population essential elements or programs of health care (NESAC 1998; MoH 1999, 2004; HMG-N and NPC 2002; Martinez and Koirala 2002). Some efforts have been made by various governments in Nepal during the successive five-year plans to improve people's health status and to enhance access to basic health care. After the multi-party system was introduced in Nepal in 1990, notable progress has been made in improving the primary health care service network by establishing primary health care centers at the electoral constituency level, sub-health post at the Village Development Committee (VDC) level, and improving the outreach services with the provision of female maternal and child health workers (MCHW), village health workers (VHW), and FCHV at the VDC level. There is some progress in improving access to water supply and sanitation, although great differences still exist between and within social groups. Immunization has shown the most dramatic improvement compared to other health programs.

However, the health status and health services available to people in rural Nepal are among the worst ever found in the modern world (Woollard 2005). Health care centers frequently lack trained personnel and medical supplies. A large segment of the population relies on traditional healers (see Chapter 4 in this book). Children are particularly vulnerable, because they are less likely to be brought long distances to health centers, and they are more prone to diseases than adults. Pneumonia and diarrhea are the two leading causes of death among children under five in Nepal.

Some demographic and health indicators of Nepal

In 2014, life expectancy at birth in Nepal was 69.6 (UNDP 2015). The most common diseases are dysentery, tuberculosis, Hepatitis, and HIV/AIDS; the most common causes of mortality are respiratory infections, coronary heart disease, stroke, and prenatal conditions. Neonatal mortality decreased from 45 per 1,000 live births in 1991–1995 to 33 per 1,000 live births in the period 2006–2010. Infant mortality has declined from 79 deaths per 1,000 live births in 1991–1995 to 33 per 1,000 deaths in 2014. Under-five mortality decreased from 118 deaths per 1,000 live births to 38 deaths per 1,000 live births in 2014 (MoHP et al. 2012; Central Bureau of Statistics 2015).

The maternal mortality ratio decreased from 539 to 170 within 15 years (UNDP 2011). Improved maternal health services have been crucial for reducing maternal and infant mortality. However, there are large differences in the use of antenatal care services between rural and urban areas, ecological zone, development regions, levels of education, and wealth. The 2011 NDHS report stated that 88 percent of mothers living in urban areas received antenatal care from a skilled provider, compared with only 55 percent of mothers in rural areas. Looking at regions in Nepal, skilled service was given to 63 percent of mothers living in the Tarai, 53 percent in the hill zone, less than

55 percent in the mid-western region, and 52 percent of mothers in the mountain zone.

Fertility in Nepal has dropped substantially over the past two decades. According to the NDHS 2011, fertility declined from 4.6 births per woman in the 1996 to 2.6 births per woman in 2011. This is due to improved communication and greater access to modern methods of contraception, extended spousal separation due to migration, changes in perception of the ideal number of children, increased age for marrying, and increased use of safe abortion services.

A birth delivered in a health facility is important for reducing death arising from complications in pregnancy. Nepal is promoting safe motherhood through initiatives such as providing financial assistance through maternal incentives schemes to women seeking skilled delivery care in a health facility. Subsidies are also provided to health institutions on the basis of deliveries conducted. NDHS 2011 showed that only 35 percent of births take place in a health facility, 26 percent are delivered in a public sector health facility, 2 percent in a nongovernment health facility, and 7 percent in a private facility. Children in urban areas are more than twice as likely (71 percent) to be delivered in an institutional setting as children born in rural areas. There is a strong association between health facility delivery, mother's education, and wealth.

According to the Mathema Commission Report 2015, there are about 24,000 hospital beds, 15,666 medical officers, 4,025 specialists, and 28,364 nurses working in Nepal. Out of 95 government hospitals, only 16 are located in rural areas all medical colleges and teaching hospitals are located in urban areas. Thus, there is a wide gap between the urban and rural areas in educational attainment, health care facilities, transportation, communication, and economic status.

Medical services in Nepal are firmly located in the broader context of the international health care market. Allopathic medicine has become a profitable commodity, promoted and marketed by multinational pharmaceutical companies, and the access for sick persons to medical services is governed by their ability to pay fees. Since the poorest are among the least healthy, market principles usually fail to match health needs and medical care (Subedi 2001). Health services has never adequately reached the masses. The health services are poor due to the weak position in policy and planning programs, poor commitment during implementation of health and related programs, disrespect for people's health rights, continuing political instability, and the lack of people's participation. There is a need to review the past, admit failures, and change policy to allow more participation by the people and their representatives from the villages upward in the decision-making processes in health care.

Health issues as elements in social development

The description of health conditions in the previous section makes it abundantly clear that we are faced with a serious social problem. This is a problem not only for each individual who suffers from malnutrition and illnesses, but also for Nepal as a country. A healthy population is Nepal's most crucial resource for social and economic development.

The term 'development' can be interpreted in different ways with implications for the choice of strategy to solve social problems, including health problems. It is common to distinguish between three development paradigms: modernization, dependency, and participatory (Melkote and Steeves 2001).

The *modernization* paradigm dominated in academic discussions and practical development work during the 1950s and 1960s. Modernization was particularly seen as something that ought to take place within autonomous Third World countries in order to bring so-called underdeveloped countries into increasingly higher levels of development. Development was defined as economic growth with rapid and sustained expansion of material production, productivity, and income per head. This would be obtained by introducing capital-intensive, but labor saving technology that could change the industrial infrastructure. It was also necessary to use communication to bring ideas, knowledge, and skills to people. The communication part was important for creating among people a positive attitude toward modernization, in other words, to create a modernization culture. This required four elements: *awareness* of the problem of underdevelopment, *knowledge* about material technology and skills, a positive *attitude* toward using new technology to cope with underdevelopment, and finally, to change people's *behavior* so they actually begin using new technology.

These four elements constitute a diffusion process described in more detail in the next section. We should also be aware of the fact that centralized planning was seen as the best way to use available resources efficiently on the road from underdevelopment toward higher levels of development. This aspect has significant implications for which parts of the population benefit from development. In Nepal, this evidently brings forth the issue of changes in urban and rural areas, in central and remote parts of the country.

The modernization paradigm emphasized the role of mass media for information dissemination in order to obtain technological and social change. High media exposure was believed to make people receptive to changing their traditional beliefs and attitudes. The modernization perspective had a tendency to blame individual as well as social constraints for underdevelopment, but it did not recognize that external constraints indeed put limits on development. These external constraints are international trade, economic imperialism of international corporations, and the vulnerability and dependency of the recipients of technical assistance programs. Moreover, the modernization paradigm failed to differentiate between the developing countries with rich resources and those with low resources. These two types of developing countries may need entirely different development strategies to achieve the best results.

After some years it became apparent that social change in many of the countries that had followed the modernization paradigm did not go in the expected direction. Therefore, in the mid-1970s, there evolved an alternative pathway to development. The *dependency* paradigm asked why development did not work in some of the developing countries. This paradigm argued that foreign aid, technology, and information created underdevelopment rather than being a force for development. This relationship implied that capital and technology were introduced from abroad by foreign governments and international organizations such as the World Bank or international nongovernment organizations (INGOs) such as the United Nations Development Programme (UNDP), the WHO, etc. In this way, the very same modernization process that should bring countries out of underdevelopment put them in a state of dependency in an economic, political, and cultural sense. Contracts about trade or for aiding specific projects created economic as well as political dependency. The transnational corporations and international trade tactics monopolized the economic scene. Foreign aid often implies that developed countries affect conditions on the political and social scene in developing countries (Mishra 1987). The dependency relationship was also described as imperialism, reflecting a situation characterized by uneven power relations.

Dependency communication theorists analyzed mass media as an 'ideological state apparatus' that reinforced the dependent character of the production relationship. The transnational corporations penetrated the political sphere via their control over modern technology, and their ideological and economic logic influenced the content of education. The advanced capitalist countries sold the most sophisticated communication technologies to less industrialized countries, and transnational corporations controlled much of the production of news and entertainment programs. The myth was created by these countries that advanced mass media technology could contribute to overcoming some of the problems of underdevelopment.

From the 1980s, the *participatory* paradigm became more pronounced. The emphasis is put on active participation of the people at the grass roots level, and the process of development is assessed as being specific for each Third World country. This means that there is no universal development strategy, but that a specific one must be designed according to each country's specific natural environments, available natural and human resources, and cultural values (Freire 1972). Everett Rogers (1995: 127) has defined the participatory paradigm in the following way:

> Development is defined as a widely participatory process of social change in a society intended to bring about both social and material advancement (including greater equality, freedom, and other valued qualities) for the majority of people through their gaining greater control over their environment.

The crucial difference between these three ways of looking at development is the degree to which people take part in decision-making processes regarding social, political, and cultural affairs. In the modernization approach, professional experts and top politicians make a list of criteria against which the level of development is measured. This is a top-down process. On the other hand, a bottom-up process means that people themselves participate in defining what the important needs are and how they should be met.

Another relevant term is 'sustainable development'. Melkote and Steeves (2001: 35) writes that this perspective "assumes that maintaining the biological diversity of the planet is essential to the survival of humanity. Hence development that does not prioritize environmental sustainability is doomed to fail." Subedi (2005: 234) looks at this type of development in a Nepalese context and describes it as process in which desirable social objectives are taken care of. It implies "help for the very poor, marginalized and disadvantaged; self-reliant development; basic health and educational facilities for all; clean water and shelter for all; human beings, in other words, are the resources in this concept." Similarly, Panday's (1999: 4) concern about Nepal's failed development was:

> not about the technical aspects of whether and how development has failed. It is about why is it that the country's precarious social

and economic condition embedded in an uncertain and probably unhelpful external milieu does not attract commensurate behavioural response from the responsible quarters. The latter includes not only the state institutions and political parties but also the various agents and institutions of what is called the civil society.

He further wrote (1999: 2): "If there is development, the average citizen of the country should feel reassured that they are in greater control over their environment and that they have a command over the range of choices available to them for their future progress." While acknowledging that the academic definition of development can be disputed, he argued that (Panday 1999: 7): "the ordinary people recognise it when they feel it and enjoy it." Improved air quality or happier children are both conditions that people will notice immediately.

According to the World Health Organization (WHO 1999) and United Nations Development Programme (UNDP 2000), human poverty, poor health, food scarcity, and malnutrition represent major obstacles to social and economic development. Therefore, initiatives aimed at battling the causes of poor health are very important. In order to make such initiatives effective and not waste money and human resources, we must distinguish between conditions that are given by nature and conditions that are created by people. It is impossible for people to stop earthquakes and volcanic eruptions, and they cannot change the harsh conditions for growing crops in high altitudes and in desert areas. Besides some technological solutions, for example, irrigation in desert areas, the only way to ease the living conditions is to migrate. But man himself has also contributed to poor living conditions. Heating with coal, exhaust from cars, industrial waste, etc. have created air and soil pollution that affect people's health. At the individual level, we know that cigarette smoking, excessive alcohol consumption, drug use, unsafe sexual relationships, and unbalanced nutrition create different types of illness.

Brief introduction to communication theory

Communication is a process in which a sender transmits a message (ideas, facts, information) to a receiver. Communication can take place directly from person to person, or it can happen through various media. During the 1930s and 1940s, mass media communication was believed to be a direct one-way process from the sender to the receiver. This was called the Stimulus–Response (S–R) model of communication. In an election study in 1940 (Lazarsfeld et al. 1948), the researchers discovered that there were one or several opinion leaders who served as mediators of a sender's message to the receivers. They were so-called gate keepers who selected information in the mass media (the sender) and transmitted it to the audience. The two-step flow model had been created. It also turned out that people did not seek just one person for information and evaluations, but that they had different opinion leaders for different topics. Thus, they talked with one particular person about local affairs, with another about fashions, and still another when they wanted to know more about foreign affairs.

The lesson to be learned from this research is that we have to decide *who* our audience comprise, that is, who the receivers of the message should be. Do we want to reach a mass audience, for instance, the inhabitants in a whole country, within a particular region, or in local areas? Or do we want to reach specific groups with particular needs? Our choice of communication medium depends on this decision. The choice of mediating form also depends on what we want to transmit (the message), and what our purpose for initiating a communication process is.

Let us first look at whom we want to reach. It can be a target population and/or a receiver group (Windahl and Signitzer 1993). A *target population* comprises those individuals whose behavior, attitudes, or knowledge we want to influence, directly or indirectly, while a *receiver group* is the group for which a certain message is intended. We can look at these two audience types in three ways. First, the target population and the receiver group can be identical. For instance, we may want to reach all members of an ethnic group with a specific message with the intention of influencing their level of knowledge, their attitudes, or their behavior. Second, the receiver group can be situated within the target population. For instance, we may want to reach all women (target population) within a particular ethnic group (receiver group). Third, the receiver group can be situated outside the target population. For instance, we may want to reach professional health workers (the receiver group) whom we hope can convey health information to a particular ethnic group or to women within a particular ethnic group (the target population).

This description of audience types also alludes to what the purpose of a communication can be. People who initiate a communication process, be it parents, teachers, politicians, business managers, etc., want to make a difference by increasing people's *awareness* of a certain issue, to change their level of *knowledge* about various aspects of the issue, to influence people's *values and attitudes* that are related to the issue, and, finally, to change people's *behavior* with respect to a specific issue. Awareness, knowledge, values, and behavior are stepping stones in a communication ladder. Thus, we cannot expect people to stop smoking if they are not aware of, or do not know about, the health risks involved. Certain values may represent an even more important obstacle to behavioral change. In this chapter we are particularly concerned with those values and attitudes that serve as significant cultural preconditions for successfully reaching specific target populations with health related information.

Any communication process includes a sender and a receiver who are sharing a message. There are several ways to look at what is going on between these two partners. We already have described the traditional *effect model* in which a message was transmitted directly from a sender to a receiver. The two-step flow and multi-step flow introduced the *diffusion model*. Diffusion is a process by which an innovation is communicated through certain channels over time among members of, for instance, a professional or occupational group, an ethnic or age group, etc. (Rogers 1995). An innovation can be an idea (e.g. reasons for a particular illness), a practice (e.g. stopping smoking to prevent lung cancer), or an object (e.g. X-ray machine) that is perceived as new by an individual or by several people. A successful diffusion process begins when people get to know about a new idea, a new practice or a new object. Then they have to be persuaded that the new thing is good before they decide to adopt the new idea, practice, or object. The final stage is when they actually have accepted the new idea or implemented a new practice or object, and that they after a while are being confirmed in their decisions.

The validity of the diffusion model was first tested within the agricultural sector. Research found that a particular group of people collected information about certain machines, seeds, fertilizers, etc., and then introduced this in their farming. These people were called the early innovators, and it could take several months or years before knowledge and technology had been diffused to most of the farmers within an area. However, once the tide turned, the curve for the number of people who adopted the new technology became very steep. When the spreading of the innovation had lasted a while (months or years) the diffusion curve flattened.

Both the effect model and the diffusion model look at the communication process as going from one or more senders to one or more receivers, to an audience. The receiver does, however, consider how relevant the message/content is for himself/herself, and selects accordingly. The discovery of the opinion leaders in the two-step flow communication process and of the early adopters in the diffusion process proved that such considerations took place.

The *participatory model* offers a totally different view of the relationship between those involved in a communication process. The participatory approach can be described as the opening of a dialogue in which the sender and the receiver interact continuously and reflect constructively about the situation, defining what their needs and problems are, and jointly discuss how needs can be met and problems can be solved, and finally, that the partners involved can actually begin to act accordingly. Participatory communication can be seen as an ideal speech situation between equal partners. It has also been called network communication. This implies that the distinction between sender, message, and receiver becomes less relevant because there is an ongoing interaction in which people share relevant information in order to reach an agreement about what the problems to be solved are, and how to do it. With Panday's (1999: 2) words: "If there is development, the average citizens of the country should feel reassured that they are in greater control over their environment and that they have a command over the range of choices available to them for their future progress."

Participatory communication is not easy to practice. It is a time-consuming process demanding patience from all people involved. Figure 7.1 shows the participatory model's complexity and will be illustrated by using people's wellbeing and health as an issue. In the figure, A would be health workers such as nurses, medical doctors, practitioners in alternative medicine, etc., while B can be people who live within a specific geographic area (a village, a region, etc.) or who belong to a particular social group (e.g. women, ethnic group, etc.). A basic prerequisite for A and B to have an interest in each other at all is that they see it worthwhile to exchange information.

But, what type of information? For instance, the WHO publishes annual reports about people's health conditions in countries throughout the world. One example in Nepal is the disability survey that Impact Nepal (1998) did in the Sindhuli District. The survey registered the frequency of the following disabilities: hearing impairment, no speech and language, visual impairment, mentally retarded, and physical disability. The percentage of disabled persons in the whole population in the Sindhuli District was 9 percent (Impact Nepal 1998: 6). Other studies have revealed a high degree of malnutrition that causes several types of illness.

Do people themselves perceive the same health problems as the professionals? Most mothers notice quickly when a child has diarrhea, but they do not always know the best way to treat it. It can be more difficult to discover – and to acknowledge – that a child is

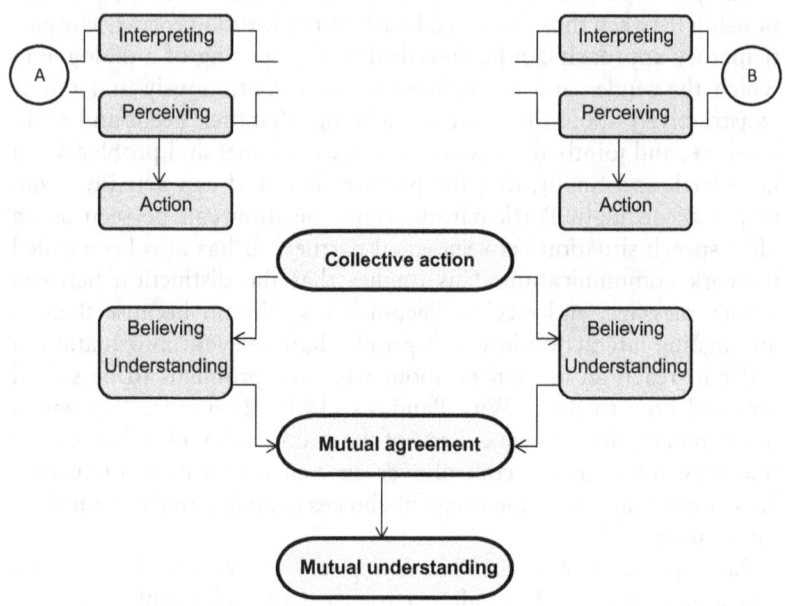

Figure 7.1 Information exchange and collective action in the participatory model

Source: Designed by and courtesy of Manohar Pradhan

mentally disabled, and almost impossible to know that this can be caused by iodine deficiency. The relationship between A and B raises two issues. People concerned (B) may not be able to interpret correctly the symptoms that professionals (A) are trained to spot and understand. Equally important is the fact that mothers may perceive symptoms and illness as caused by fate (*karma*) and/or evil spirits. Thus, the information that A and B can exchange is obtained within different cultural contexts. This means that the very same facts are interpreted and perceived differently by A and B, respectively. Therefore, we must be prepared to spend much time to identify what people (B) regard as problematic for their wellbeing. It is not sufficient to approach mothers with a rational explanation that iodine deficiency causes mental disability.

To initiate some kind of action may be one possible step forward. For instance, based on knowledge that zinc supplement can treat diarrhea,

Norwegian doctors started a project in the late 1990s inviting mothers to bring their sick children to a clinic in Bhaktapur. Eventually the medical team managed to persuade mothers in the area to come regularly to the clinic to be trained in giving their child a drop of zinc. It took not long before the number of children with diarrhea decreased. Action had proved that there was some truth in what the medical team told them. By inviting the mothers to come to the clinic, they met other women and could see that they had a common problem. The Norwegian team trained Nepalese health workers who, it was hoped, could inspire the women for collective action in the neighborhood, that is, to continue with the zinc supplement if the diarrhea returned. Eventually the women would understand the relationship between zinc and the absence of an illness, and thus believe in the importance of giving their children this particular supplement. By participating actively in this process, health workers and indigenous women had reached a mutual agreement and a mutual understanding. The challenge in such initiatives is to assure that the behavioral change lasts over a longer period of time.

There are four factors that can influence people's willingness to enter into a participatory communication process. First, they must believe that the facts they are presented are *true*. In other words, when the mothers saw that a repeated drop of zinc healed their children's diarrhea, the chances of them accepting this relationship as true increased. Second, people must see the *relevance* of a new idea or technique. This was probably the most important reason why the medical team managed to persuade women in Bhaktapur to come to the clinic in the first place; their children's health was at stake. Third, communication initiatives must be perceived as being *sincere* and serving people's own interests. Development aid and medical research can be problematic in this respect. Time-limited projects, be it in charge of national or foreign agencies, are done with good intentions. At the same time we must acknowledge that also professional prestige can be involved, for instance in a medical research project. However, the crucial aspect of any innovation process is to transfer knowledge to the people who live in a neighborhood, in a village or in a region. Again with Panday's (1999: 3) words:

> Admittedly, there are instances of genuine accomplishments due to the enterprising efforts of some individuals or groups. But we cannot accept them as symbolic of 'development', if they do not have the property of being a part of a cumulative, inter-linked, sustained, and socially inclusive process.

Thus, 'good intentions' should not mean just doing something for people, but rather that people are given resources (knowledge, techniques, equipment, etc.) that can enable them to be in charge themselves of improving their living conditions.

The fourth factor affecting people's trust in a participatory communication process is *comprehensibility*. People must understand what is going on; that an innovation has implications for whatever their problems may be, and that they understand how to use new technology.

At the individual or group level we must be aware of the character of the social relationship between those who know (A) and those who do not know (B). Two types of information are exchanged between A and B: *content* information and *relationship* information (Kreps 1990). Content information includes facts, for instance, about the nature of health, reasons for different illnesses, and health care. On the other hand, relationship information conveys the level of concern, sensitivity, and power that health workers express toward patients, and that health educators show during meetings with people (their audience). To be aware of this distinction is crucial for a participatory communication process to succeed. Health workers can be professionally excellent and score high on content information, but they fail dismally to get people involved because their relationship information indicates that people (e.g. women in a village) are not regarded as equal partners when defining what the problem may be as well as deciding the best way to solve it.

In order to understand the communication process between health workers (A) and people (B), we must know something about the cultural preconditions that each part brings into the relationship. Culture implies health beliefs with respect to four questions (Subedi 2001): (1) Why does this happen?, (2) Why does this happen to me?, (3) What can or should be done?, and (4) Who knows, and who can be trusted?

The first question addresses the causes for an illness. On the one hand, rational school medicine looks for physical, social, or material circumstances. Many people have the same opinion about the reasons for good health, but we also know that beliefs in fate (*karma*) and evil spirits still exist (Chapter 3 in this book, "Illness Causation and Interpretation in a Newari Town," looks closer at this issue). Such attitudes must be treated seriously in a participatory communication process. Culture can also offer explanations to why just a particular person or a particular social group is afflicted. An evil spirit aims at one person in particular, while zinc deficiency is a general phenomenon among children in many parts of Nepal. This illustrates a cultural difference between a personal, irrational oriented explanation, and a rational nutrition-oriented explanation. Depending on the cultural beliefs, there are also different answers to the third question. An explanation based on fate or evil spirits asks for supernatural treatment, while the rational explanation implies treatment according to the principles of school medicine. This naturally leads to two different choices regarding whom to turn to for treatment, the shaman, the healer, or the medical doctor (Subedi 2003).

Access is a prerequisite for development communication where people participate in programs for social change. Availability of mass media in a country or specific community, however, does not guarantee that people will use media. A multi-channel approach for development communication would ensure a wider reach with lasting effect.

Communication and social change

The previous sections have made it clear that the purpose for initiating a communication process is to obtain changes in ideas, knowledge, attitudes, and behavior. When businesses spend much money on advertising, the goal is to persuade more people to buy certain products. Another example is when private and government agencies want to allure tourists by printing catalogues and paying for advertisements in national and international mass media. Also voluntary associations depend on communication to reach members with information and to recruit new members, and teachers communicate with their students. In other words, communication is an integrated part of social life.

Our concern is how communication can be used to cope with social problems, and to focus on Nepal in particular. We have already emphasized the distinction between objective and subjective definitions of social problems. We must also keep in mind that there may be different conceptions of social change and development, as expressed by Mishra (1987: 105):

> Development is somehow holy, uplifting and attractive. It is, however, also mysterious. The object is subjectively perceived and the totality of subjectivities does not add up to an objective description and/or assessment.

We also have argued for a participatory communication approach in which people's subjective views are crucial. This does not mean, however, that objective data and indexes should be ignored. This type of statistics actually enables us to compare across countries and to identify the particular social problems in the country we are interested in

(Chapter 9 in this book offers one illustration). The participatory element becomes relevant once we reach the stage when we are ready to approach a special group of people.

What are, then, the social problems in Nepal? UNDP's annual reports on human development in about 170 countries in the world offer information about human wellbeing, not just economic trends, and form the basis for calculating a Human Development Index (HDI). The three basic dimensions in this index are (UNDP 2000: 240):

- A long and healthy life, as measured by life expectancy at birth.
- Knowledge, as measured by the adult literacy rate and the combined primary, secondary and tertiary gross enrolment ratio.
- A decent standard of living, as measured by Gross National Product (GNP) per capita.

Depending on how countries score on this index, they are classified as having high, medium, or low human development. According to the latest UNDP Report (2015), Nepal's HDI was 0.548, placing Nepal among the world's 15 poorest countries. In comparison, the HDI for Norway was 0.944, for Great Britain 0.907, and for India 0.609.

Safe drinking water and toilet facilities are important elements for good health and public sanitation. Generally, tap water, tube-wells, and covered wells are regarded as safe or improved sources of water, and it is assumed that there is low probability of contamination. According to the 2011 Nepal Census, 48.1 percent of the households used tap water, and 35.3 percent tube-wells as their usual drinking water sources. Similarly, 61.6 percent of the households had toilet facilities and about two-third of them were using flush toilet (Kayastha 2015). Thus, a fair number of the population does not use toilets, and those who do use toilets do not have sufficient infrastructure of public sewerage facilities where they live.

It is beyond any doubt that health workers and health administrators have a challenging job. Although this chapter focuses on health and communication, it is worth repeating that not all social problems are communication problems. For instance, in the introduction we quoted Brundtland (1999: viii) who emphasized the close relationship between poor health and poverty. There are, however, many reasons why people are poor. For instance, natural factors can cause harsh environments for growing crops in high altitude areas in Nepal, or they can create draughts in desert areas in Africa, and people can be poor because the distribution of resources, including income, is unequal. This is a political matter that requires that citizens mobilize in order to influence political decisions to change their life situation. Communication is a crucial tool for political mobilization, but this chapter does not delve any further into this. We shall move on to look at other reasons for poor health and particular diseases, and to what extent communication can contribute to solve health problems.

This is not the place for describing strictly medical explanations for poor health. Although they are important for health workers' choice of treatment, we are more interested in general factors that can cause diseases. In addition to poverty, illness can be caused by malnutrition (Aase 2002; Andersen 2002), infections (e.g. from the malaria insect), lifestyle (e.g. smoking, too much alcohol and fat food), poor sanitation, and polluted environment. These conditions can be attacked at a structural and/or at an individual level. At the structural level, politicians may decide to establish welfare programs to reduce poverty. Malnutrition can be reduced with programs for food supplements, and malaria can be fought by distributing bed-nets and medicine, and also by cultivating malaria-rich marshes. Restrictions on advertising from the tobacco industry and information about the health risks related to smoking may change people's behavior. Regulations regarding the use of private and public vehicles and industries in cities may improve air quality that, in turn, reduces the amount of respiratory problems. At the individual level education is the key to coping with all these health problems – education and some money.

Thus health problems can be approached by looking at health-*directed* factors (medical) and/or factors in people's life situation that are deemed to be health *related* in the sense that they affect people's wellbeing in one way or another. Available health facilities, material infrastructure such as clean water, sanitation, pollution, etc., and health information are all health related factors. The Ottawa Charter (1986: 1) defined health promotion in the following way:

> Health promotion is the process of enabling people to increase control over, and to improve, their health. To reach a state of complete physical, mental and social well-being, and individuals or groups must be able to identify and to realize aspirations, to satisfy needs, and change or cope with the environment. Health is, therefore, seen as a resource for everyday life, not the objective of living. Health is a positive concept emphasizing social and personal resources, as well as physical capacities. Therefore, health promotion is not just the responsibility of the health sector, but goes beyond healthy life-styles to wellbeing.

The Ottawa Charter listed five means to promote action for improved health:

- Building healthy public policy.
- Creating supportive environments.
- Strengthening community action.
- Reorienting health services.
- Developing personal skills and self-efficacy, that is people's assessment of their own ability to enact recommended behavior.

These quotes from the Ottawa Charter give a short version of the importance of getting people involved in projects aimed at improving their social conditions, health included. We also must discuss to what extent changes in the type of structural elements listed in the Ottawa Charter are needed. For instance, to persuade the government in a country to invest in health facilities may require pressure from international organizations such as WHO and UNDP. It also would be beneficial if the politicians acknowledged that they have something to gain politically by spending money on health provisions (Justice 1986).

Over time, many guides and handbooks have described ways to plan and implement a strategy for health communication (e.g. Haaland et al. 2001). The Center for Communication Programs, Johns Hopkins School of Public Health in the USA, is regarded as one of the top institutions for testing health communication material. In *Health Communication*, Phyllis T. Piotrow and colleagues (1997) focused on family planning and reproductive health. This is, of course, a crucial issue in health policy and practical work, but the book is also relevant for other aspects of people's health. It combines theoretical reflections with descriptions of how different types of communication material have been tested and evaluated, and it describes five steps for designing a strategy for health communication aimed at enhancing social development: (1) Setting objectives, (2) Positioning, (3) Assessing communication strategies, (4) Assessing implementing organizations, (5) Documentation and evaluation.

Setting objectives

It is important to spend some time on the first step. We have already stated that successful communication requires that we must decide whom we want to reach with a specific message. We also have seen that the 'who' in the communication process can be people who define health policy objectives at the national level, in specific areas, or among specific population groups. Programs to accomplish our goals depend on whom we want to reach. Piotrow et al. (1997: 59) mention "high quality of health care, more integrated reproductive health services, or economic sustainability over time." The time element is important (ibid.: 60):

> Long-term vision can set bold objectives. [. . .] Every program needs a long-term vision. It can empower people because it shows what is important. It can stimulate teamwork because it shows what everyone needs to do. And it can strengthen organization because it generates new energy.

So many programs have failed because public health officials or political leaders want quick results without having to spend too many resources. Communication objectives should be SMART (ibid.: 63):

S   Specific – defining what is to be accomplished in terms of specific steps to behavioral change among specific, well-defined audiences.
M   Measurable – quantifying the objectives by indicating a numerical or percentage change expected.
A   Appropriate – defining intended changes that are culturally and locally acceptable.
R   Realistic – avoiding objectives that are beyond the scope of available resources, contrary to relevant experience, or unrelated to communication efforts.
T   Time bound – identifying the time frame in which changes should be achieved.

It may be difficult to measure in numerical terms the changes we want to obtain. However, some kind of change should be defined before we start planning a time-consuming communication process. For instance, we should know whether we want to reach the whole population – a mass audience – or specific groups, either as receiver group or target group as described previously.

Positioning

The term 'positioning' comes from the commercial world and its strategic implication is to present (Piotrow et al. 1997: 64) "an issue, service, or product in such a way that it stands out from other comparable or competing issues, services, or products and is appealing and persuasive."

The point with positioning is that people should become aware of, and understand, the purpose of a particular program. This can be obtained by the use of a certain terminology or images. In countries with high illiteracy rates, images have proved to be a very effective way to create awareness about health issues (Haaland et al. 2001). Positioning must take cultural values into consideration. Piotrow et al. (1997: 67) illustrates this by describing many western nations' emphasis on individual human rights in contrast to the Chinese political system's focus on national interests. For instance, political leaders in China have promoted family planning as a patriotic duty. The answers to health related questions also depend on people's cultural context (Subedi 2001). This aspect of culture must be taken into consideration also in the positioning phase.

Assessing communication strategies

To assess communication strategies requires a discussion of which steps to take at different phases. We cannot expect anything but failure if we tell mothers that zinc supplement is good for their children before a system for making the supplement available has been established. Thus, the clinic in Bhaktapur was set up with a medical team and a training program for Nepalese health workers before they told people in the neighborhood about the program. It also might be worthwhile to consider whether to launch a nation-wide campaign or to begin communicating to small groups.

The PABASA program in the Philippines (Solon 1999) is an excellent example of a communication design that begins with a small group and expands to whole villages. First, a team of nutrition experts from the Nutrition Center of the Philippines (NCP) got permission from the village chairperson to invite about ten women – who were seen as opinion leaders – to a two-day meeting about nutrition, healthy food, sanitation, etc. These women afterwards formed other groups, and the process continued until, if all went well, the new information had reached all households in the village. The PABASA program also illustrates a multimedia approach by using informal discussions, games, brochures, posters, and information about nutrition given by the local store keeper. Campaigns in mass media such as television and radio can be effective to raise awareness among a large audience, but other mediating forms seem to be better if we also want behavioral change.

We often perceive health information as very serious. The content in health communication is indeed serious, but serious information can be presented in an entertaining way. Research has shown (Piotrow et al. 1997: 76; Storey 1999) that popular songs, television series, soap operas, and theatrical performances in the village square increase people's curiosity about health issues. Apparently it is also easier to remember facts that have been presented in an entertaining form and not as plain facts. This is particularly important when the audience is young people. Research (e.g. Green et al. 2002) indicates that hard facts about health related behavior may be ignored by adolescents because they are risk takers. They simply do not believe that 'this can happen to me', and besides, it is exciting to challenge their luck.

Finally, communication strategies should be designed in such a way that the information is given by credible sources (people and/or institutions) that are trusted and respected by the audience we want to reach (Piotrow et al. 1997: 81).

Assessing implementing organizations

The next step is to make a plan for implementing the communication strategy we have designed. Who will do it, and how to do it, are the two crucial issues at this stage. Health communication requires resources that organizations, and not individuals, can provide. (Piotrow et al. 1997: 84) write: "The major criteria for implementing organizations are competence, commitment, clout, and continuity."

The previously described projects in Bhaktapur and the Philippines (Solon 1999) were run by organizations that sent people with a professional training into the field. Particularly the PABASA project illustrates a participatory approach in which women in local communities were treated as equal partners in bringing nutrition and health information throughout the village. Community participation is often crucial for health communication to succeed (Cohen 1996).

There is one problem with using professionals in health communication. Previously, the chapter distinguished between content information and relationship information (Kreps 1990). Aubel and Niang (1991) made a study of midwives' interpersonal communication behavior during family planning consultations in Senegal. They found that some of the consultations did not go well because the midwives had a top-down 'I-know-best' attitude toward their clients. Thus the women did not fully receive or acknowledge the objectively correct content information because they perceived the relationship information negatively. The study's recommendation was (Aubel and Niang 1991: 79):

> From the beginning to the end of the family planning consultation the midwives should involve the client in a dialogue in which the

client is encouraged to ask questions, and is asked her opinion in terms of decisions to be made and follow-up action to be taken.

Documentation and evaluation

The last, but not least important, step in Piotrow and colleagues' communication strategy is documentation and evaluation. Everything we do from setting objectives to implementing a communication strategy must be documented. What are our goals, what type of change in awareness, knowledge, attitudes, and behavior do we want to obtain? Which group of people do we want to reach with health information? How can we best communicate to our receiver group and target group? And how are we going to implement the communication strategy we have agreed upon? It is only such detailed documentation that enables us to evaluate if we have reached our goals, or if we are on the right track.

Cultural preconditions

Although culture is a slippery concept we nevertheless cannot be without it. In a general sense, culture includes beliefs, values, feelings, symbols and meanings, food, and modes of social interaction (White 1999; Subedi 2004). Human beings orient themselves in space and time by means of language and social relations; with the body, food, and clothes; by the structure of everyday life; and in terms of symbols and frameworks provided by public myth, religion, and rituals (Delaney 2004). It is important to dig deeper and analyze both the particular meaning embodied in these phenomena and the way they are interconnected. If we try to give health education to a specific group of people with the purpose to change their existing practices, it is important to know their total way of life and how they perceive it. This helps us to understand them better and to assess the best way forward to change their behavior. This is illustrated in this book's Chapter 5 on food, health, and illness ideology in the Nepalese town Kirtipur. However, it is extremely important to investigate the ways in which power (aggression, repression, and exploitation) influences cultural expressions.

The overview in Table 7.1 enables us to compare cultural expressions among women in five different ethnic groups in Nepal. It shows the terms used locally by the mothers to describe ARI and illnesses among children. It seems very clear that mothers from different ethnic backgrounds use different words (language) to indicate the similar type of signs and symptoms. In order to understand the case history

Table 7.1 Terms and expression to describe pneumonia and danger symptoms

Brahman/ Chhetri	Tamang	Tharu	Musahar	Muslim
Swah swah garne/Chhito chhito swash ferne (fast breathing)	Kokha hanne (chest in-drawing)	Jar aune (fever)	Aankha munne (stare for a long time)	Jukam, Thandi, Bhukar (cough, cold, fever)
Ghyar ghyar garne (noisy breathing)	Ghyar ghyar garne (noisy breathing)	Khokee lagne (cough)	Naak sur sur karche (breathing problem)	Naak sur sur karche (breathing problem)
Saas pherna garo (difficulty in breathing)	Na nabha khaji (unable to cough out mucous)	Swah swah garne (difficult breathing)	Ghanti ghar ghar karche (noisy breathing)	Pajra marchel Khapche (chest in drawing)
Kokha hanne (chest in-drawing)	Ghanti sar sar lazi (noisy breathing)	Aaama ko dudh khana nasakne (unable to suckle)	Neta ayeche (unable to cough out, mucous)	Bachha roiche (cry all the time)
Dum phulne (swollen breathing)	Na khaji (mucous flow)	Kokha dumaiche (chest pain)	Dudh nakhayeche (unable to suckle)	Ma ke dudh nakhaiche (unable to suckle)
Chhat pataune (restlessness)	Nodpa (cough)	Dulki jar (shivering fever)	Cup bhaelache (cough)	Ultiaaune (vomiting)
Salang Sulung Hune (weakness/ convulsion)	Jar khaji (fever)	Ghanti ghar ghar karchhe (noisy breathing)	Thandi lagaiche (cold)	Bhukh nai lagichhe (no appetite)
Sarir/Nidhar tato hune (increased body temperature)	Aankhami (unable to eat)	Dublaidai jane (weight loss)	Ulti aune (vomiting)	
Nasutne (unable to sleep)	Po boba (swollen stomach)	Dhekarwa (convulsions)	Paanj mariche (chest in drawing)	
Sutirahane (too sleepy)	Simbatu khaji (cold sweat)	Rune (cry incessantly)	Chatpat garne (restlessness)	
Khana kam khane (loss of appetite)	Nepale/ Mastira lagyo (pneumonia)		Bachha roiche (cry all the time)	
Dudh nakahane (don't feel like suckling)	Dudha khana nasakne (unable to swallow)		Bhundi tala mathi jane (strong movement of stomach)	
			Pajra khapche (chest in-drawing)	
			Lamo lamo sans pherne (difficulty in breathing)	

Source: Subedi (2006)

of a sick child, it is necessary to know the terms expressed by mothers within different ethnic groups.

To improve people's health condition we must explore the existing health seeking behaviors within and between the groups (Helman 1990). Accessibility, availability, and accountability of the health facilities and health care practitioners affect people's search among different health facilities and health care practitioners. Also the cost of such facilities is, of course, a very important factor for their choice of healers, as illustrated in this book's second chapter.

Implication for the communication strategy

Health communication encompasses the study and use of communication strategies to inform and influence individual and community decisions that enhance good health. Health communication can contribute to disease prevention and health promotion, and is relevant in a number of contexts, including patient–practitioner relations, individual's exposure to search for, and use of, health information, the construction of public health messages and campaigns, risk communication, images of health in the mass media, and the culture at large. It also can educate consumers about how to gain access to public health facilities, to know about different aspects of the health care system, including telemedicine applications. Health communication contributes to health promotion and disease prevention in several areas through training of health professionals and patients in effective communication skills.

For individuals, effective health communication may help to raise awareness of risks and solutions to health problems, provide the motivations and skills needed to reduce these risks, and help to find support from other people in similar situations. It also can increase demand for appropriate health services and decrease demand for inappropriate health services. It can provide information to facilitate complex choices, such as selecting health plans, care providers, and treatments. For the community, health communication can be used to influence the public agenda, advocate for policies and programs, promote positive changes in the socio-economic and physical environment, improve the delivery of public health and health care services, and encourage social norms that benefit health and quality of life.

Another strategy is to distribute health messages through public education campaigns aimed at encouraging healthy behavior, creating awareness, changing attitudes, and facilitating individuals to adopt prescribed behavior. Effective health communication is a crucial precondition to obtain focus on the key health improvement activities.

The promotion of healthy behaviors, such as regular physical activity (physiotherapy or yoga), reading and sleeping habits, healthy and nutritious food, healthy weight, and safe and responsible sexual behavior, require a range of information, education, and advocacy efforts.

Health communication alone, however, cannot change systemic health related problems, such as poverty, environmental degradation, or lack of access to health care services. However, comprehensive health communication programs should include a systemic exploration of all the factors that contribute to health and of the strategies that can be used to influence these factors. Well-designed health communication activities help individuals to better understand their own and their communities' needs so that they can take appropriate actions to maximize health.

Note

1 A version of this chapter originally appeared as 'Communication Aspects in Health Care Work in Nepal', *Dhaulagiri Journal of Sociology and Anthropology*, 2: 65–100, 2008. Used with permission.

References

Aase, Tor Halfdan. 2002. "Micronutrients and Ethnicity of Diet in Arun Valley." In Ram P. Chaudhary et al., eds., *Vegetation and Society: Their Interaction in the Himalayas*, pp. 137–148. Kathmandu: Tribhuvan University and Bergen: University of Bergen.

Andersen, Peter. 2002. "Geographical Approaches to Micronutrient Deficiencies in Himalaya." In Ram P. Chaudhary et al., eds., *Vegetation and Society: Their Interaction in the Himalayas*, pp. 137–148. Kathmandu: Tribhuvan University and Bergen: University of Bergen.

Aubel, Judi and Aminata Niang. 1991. "Health Workers' Attitudes Can Create Communication Barriers." *World Health Forum* 12: 466–471.

Brundtland, Gro Harlem. 1999. "Message for the Director-General." In World Health Organization, *Making a Difference: The World Health Report*. Geneva: WHO.

Central Bureau of Statistics. 2015. *Nepal Multiple Indicator Cluster Survey 2014, Key Findings*. Kathmandu: Central Bureau of Statistics and UNICEF Nepal.

Cohen, Sylvie I. 1996. "Mobilizing Communities for Participation and Empowerment." In Jan Servaes et al., eds., *Participatory Communication for Social Change, Chapter 13*. New Delhi, Thousand Oaks and London: Sage Publications.

Delaney, Carol. 2004. *Investigating Culture: An Experiential Introduction to Anthropology*. Oxford: Blackwell Publishing.

Dixit, Hemang. 1999. *The Quest for Health*. Kathmandu: Educational Enterprise (P) Ltd.

Freire, Paulo. 1972. *Pedagogy of the Oppressed*. Harmondsworth: Penguins.

Greene, Kathryn et al. 2002. "Elaboration in Processing Adolescent Health Messages: The Impact of Egocentrism and Sensation Seeking on Message Processing." *Journal of Communication* 52(4): 812–831.

Haaland, Ane et al. 2001. *Reporting with Pictures: A Concept Paper for Researchers and Health Policy Decision-Makers*. Geneva: UNDP, World Bank and WHO.

Helman, Cecil. 1990. "Cultural Factors in Health and Illness." In Brian R. McAvoy and Liam J. Donaldson, eds., *Health Care for Asians*, pp. 17–27. Oxford, New York and Tokyo: Oxford University Press.

HMG-N and NPC. 2002. *Tenth Plan (2002–2007)*. Kathmandu: His Majesty's Government, National Planning Commission.

Impact Nepal. 1998. *Disability Survey in Sindhuli District, Nepal: Report*. Kathmandu: Impact Nepal.

Justice, Judith. 1986. *Policies, Plans & People: Culture and Health Development in Nepal*. Berkeley, Los Angeles and London: University of California Press.

Kayastha, Rabi Prasad. 2015. "Household Amenities and Durable Goods." In *Population Monograph of Nepal*, Vol. 3, pp. 243–284. Kathmandu: GoN, NPC and Central Bureau of Statistics.

Kreps, Gary L. 1990. "Communication and Health Education." In Eileen Berlin Ray and Lewis Donohew, eds., *Communication and Health Systems and Applications*. Hillsdale, NJ: Lawrence Erlbaum Associates Publishers.

Lazarsfeld, Paul et al. 1948 [1944]. *The People's Choice: How the Voter Makes Up His Mind in a Presidential Campaign*. New York: Columbia University Press.

Martinez, Esperanza and Hari Koirala. 2002. *Primary Health Care Services in Nepal*. Kathmandu: USAID.

Melkot, Srinivas R. and H. Leslie Steeves. 2001. *Communication for Development in the Third World: Theory and Practice for Empowerment*. 2nd Edition. New Delhi: Sage publications.

Mishra, Chaitanya. 1987. "Development and Underdevelopment: A Preliminary Sociological Perspective (105–35)." In *Occasional Papers in Sociology and Anthropology* 1. Kathmandu: Central Department of Sociology and Anthropology, Tribhuvan University.

MoH. 1999. *Second Long-Term Health Plan*. Kathmandu: Ministry of Health.

MoH. 2004. *Vulnerable Community Development Plan for Nepal Health Sector Program Implementation Plan*. Kathmandu: Health Sector Reform Unit, Planning Division, Ministry of Health.

MoHP, New ERA, and ICF International Inc. 2012. *Nepal Demographic and Health Survey 2011*. Kathmandu: MoHP, New ERA, and ICF International Inc.

NESAC. 1998. *Nepal Human Development Report 1998*. Kathmandu: NESAC (Nepal South Asia Centre).

Ottawa Charter for Health Promotion. 1986. Report of the International Conference on Health Promotion. Geneva: WHO.

Panday, Devendra Raj. 1999. *Nepal's Failed Development: Reflections on the Mission and the Maladies*. Kathmandu: Nepal South Asia Centre.

Piotrow, Phyllis Tilson et al. 1997. "Strategic Design" Chapter 4. In *Health Communication: Lessons from Family Planning and Reproductive Health*. Westport, CT and London: Praeger.

Rogers, Everett M. 1995 [1962]. *Diffusion of Innovations* (4th Edition). New York: The Free Press.

Solon, Florentino S. et. al. 1999. *Strategies for Improving Manageability and Sustainability of Community-based Nutrition Programs*. Manila: Nutrition Center of the Philippines.

Storey, J. Douglas. 1999. "Popular Culture, Discourse, and Development: Rethinking Entertainment-Education from a Participatory Perspective." In T. Jacobsen and J. Servaes, eds., *Theoretical Approaches to Participatory Communication*, pp. 337–358. Cresskill, NJ: Hampton Press.

Subedi, Madhusudan Sharma. 2001. *Medical Anthropology of Nepal*. Kathmandu: Udaya Books.

Subedi, Madhusudan Sharma. 2003. "Healer Choice in Medically Pluralistic Cultural Settings: An Overview of Nepali Medical Pluralism." *Occasional Papers in Sociology and Anthropology* 8: 128–158.

Subedi, Madhusudan Sharma. 2004. "Indigenous Knowledge and Health Development in Nepal: An Anthropological Inquiry." *Manav Samaj* (June 2004): 135–151.

Subedi, Madhusudan Sharma. 2005. "Foreign Aid, Sustainable Development and Rapti IRDP." *Occasional Papers in Sociology and Anthropology* 9: 231–257. Kathmandu: Central Department of Sociology and Anthropology, Tribhuvan University.

Subedi, Madhusudan Sharma. 2006. "Indigenous Knowledge of Acute Respiratory Infections Management among Different Caste/Ethnic Groups in Nepal." *Education and Development*. Special issue, 22: 117–129.UNDP. 2000. *Human Development Report 2000*. New York and Oxford: Oxford University Press.

UNDP. 2011. *The Millennium Development Goals Report 2011*. Kathmandu: UNDP.

UNDP. 2015. *Human Development Report 2015*. New York: UNDP.

White, Kate. 1999. "The Importance of Sensitivity to Culture in Development Work." In Thomas Jacobsen and Jan Servaes, eds., *Theoretical Approaches to Participatory Communication*, pp. 17–49. Cresskill, NJ: Hampton Press.

Windahl, Sven and Benno Signitzer. 1993. *Using Communication Theory: An Introduction to Planned Communication*. London: Sage Publications.

Woollard, Robert. 2005. *Feasibility Study for the Proposed Patan University of Health Sciences (PUHS)*. Kathmandu: Medical School Steering Committee.

World Health Organization. 1999. *Making a Difference*. The World Health Report. Geneva: WHO.

8 Challenges to measure and compare disability

A methodological concern[1]

'Disability' is an umbrella term denoting impairments, activity limitations, and participation restrictions. Disability is a major public health issue, denoting the negative aspects of the relationship between an individual's health condition and her/his environmental and personal factors. The number of people with disability is growing due to increased life expectancy at birth and that elderly people have a higher risk of disability. The global increase in chronic health conditions such as diabetes, cardiovascular disease, cancer, and mental health disorders are associated with higher risk of disability.

Patterns of disability are influenced by trends in health conditions, as well as by environmental and other factors such as road traffic accidents, natural disasters, armed conflicts, dietary habits and patterns, physical exercise, and substance abuse, etc. Disability can be measured in different ways, affecting both the number of incidences and distribution on various variables. People with disability experience poorer levels of health than the general population, lower educational achievements, less economic participation, higher rates of poverty, and participation restrictions (WHO and the World Bank 2011).

This chapter focuses on the causes of variations in disability rates in censuses and surveys. Censuses and surveys take various approaches to measuring disability, resulting in different disability rates within the same country. The chapter also looks at thematic issues in disability data in Nepal obtained in censuses and surveys. It is important to both note that definitional issues underlie some of the difficulties in statistical analysis, and also to understand the conceptual questions shaping the efforts of those working in the various fields relating to disability. 'Disability' is a relative term, relying on the interpretation of 'normal activity' and summarizing a great number of different functional limitations occurring in any population. People may be disabled by physical, intellectual, or sensory impairment; medical conditions; or mental illness. Such impairments, conditions, or illnesses may be permanent or transitory in nature.

In 1976, the WHO operationalized three different terms – 'impairment', 'disability', and 'handicap'. Impairment is any loss or abnormality of psychological, physiological, or anatomical structure. Disability is any restriction or lack (resulting from an impairment) of ability to perform an activity in the manner or within the range of what is considered to be normal for a human being. Handicap is a disadvantage for an individual, resulting from impairment or a disability, which prevents the fulfillment of a role that is considered normal (depending on age, sex, social, and cultural factors) for that individual. In 1980, the WHO reaffirmed this classification (WHO 1980) and, in 2001, issued the International Classification of Functioning, Disability and Health (ICF). The ICF distinguishes between body function and body structures (WHO 2002).

The activists who are working for the disabled or disabled argue that impairment refers to physical or cognitive limitations that an individual may have, such as the inability to walk or speak. In contrast, disability also may refer to socially imposed restrictions, that is, the system of social constraints that are imposed on those with impairments by the discriminatory practices of society.

In many cases, the language used in certain contexts becomes critical in shaping and reflecting thoughts, beliefs, feelings, and concepts (Ellis and Kent 2011). Some words by their very nature degrade and diminish people with a disability. The phrase 'disabled young person' tends to convey a message that the only thing worth mentioning about a person is her/his disability. It is better to say 'young person with a disability' as this emphasizes the person first without denying the reality of the disability. Sometimes people with a disability are compared to normal people. This implies that the person with a disability is abnormal, and it ignores the fact that everyone has her/his own unique identity and abilities.

Defining disability

Disability data do not reflect the full extent of disability prevalence. The limitation is due partly to the conceptual framework adopted, the scope and coverage of the survey undertaken, as well as the definition, classification, and the methodology used for disability data collection.

Disability has often been defined as a physical, mental, or psychological condition that limits a person's activities. It has different meanings to different people, and in different contexts. The Global Burden of Disease (GBD) uses the term disability to refer to loss of health, where health is conceptualized in terms of functioning capacity in a set of health domains such as mobility, cognition, hearing, and vision (WHO 2004).

In the past, disability was interpreted according to a medical model, linking it to various medical conditions, and viewing it as a problem residing solely in the affected individual, resulting in an individual's inability to function (Mont 2007a). Interventions usually included medical rehabilitation and the provision of social assistance. The medical model of disability views the body as a machine to be fixed in order to come to a normal state. The line of analysis which derives from viewing disability as a purely medical condition creates a deficit in an individual, rather than changing his/her functional status; a status that affects a person's life depending on the environment he/she lives in (Mont 2007b). The relationship in the medical model is this (Hutchison 1995):

Disease or disorder → Impairment → Disability → Handicap

Once a person starts to suffer from a disease or disorder, she/he loses the normality of a psychological, physiological, or anatomical function. Due to her/his disability, a person's ability to perform expected human activity is restricted or totally absent. She/he is categorized as a disadvantaged or handicapped person that limits or prevents fulfillment of expected social roles. The concept *normalization* becomes popular as part of the medical model, and establishing curative services is regarded as the main way to make a person as normal as possible.

The medical model has been criticized by sociologists, anthropologists, human rights activists, and also by the disabled people themselves. Disabled people want acceptance in society and therefore reject being defined as abnormal. The social model conceptualizes disability as arising from the interaction of a person's functional status with the physical, cultural, and policy environments. If the environment is designed for the full range of human functioning, incorporating appropriate accommodations and support, people with functional limitations would not be 'disabled' in the sense that they would be able to fully participate in society.

The social model highlights disability as the outcome of the interaction between a person and her/his environment and, therefore, being neither person nor environment specific. The ICF, developed by the WHO (2002), is the starting point for recent developments in measuring functional capacity, and disability is increasingly seen as a multidimensional condition encompassing a wide range of physical and cognitive problems that are difficult to categorize and measure. The

ICF listed nine broad domains of functioning: learning and applying knowledge; general tasks and demands; communication; mobility; self-care; domestic life; interpersonal interaction and relationships; major life areas; and community, social, and civic life (WHO 2002). The ICF was officially endorsed by all 91 WHO member states at the 54th World Health Assembly on May 22, 2001.

The social model does not negate the worth of medical and rehabilitation services for persons with disabilities. It does, however, caution against the over-medicalization of their problems. In the social model, persons with disabilities are holders of rights, being entitled to advocate for the removal of institutional, physical, informational, and attitudinal barriers in society (UN-ESCAP 2010). The advocates of the social model argue that the interventions should be taken not only at the individual level (e.g. medical rehabilitation), but also at the societal level, for example by introducing designs to make infrastructure more accessible, providing inclusive education systems, and creating community awareness programs to combat stigma. This is at the heart of disabled people's current fight for civil and political rights. As the Convention on the Rights of Persons with Disabilities took effect on May 3, 2008, the social model of disability is gaining importance in awareness raising, policy actions, and the empowerment of persons with disabilities around the world.

The issue of comparable data

Disability is a complex multidimensional phenomenon that poses challenges for measurement. Approaches to measure disability vary across countries and influence the result. Operational measures of disability vary according to the purpose and application of the data, the conception of disability, the aspects of disability examined (impairment, activity limitations, participation restrictions, related health conditions, environmental factors), the definitions, question design, reporting sources, data collection methods, and expectations of functioning (WHO and the World Bank 2011).

The problems related to defining disability make it difficult to collect data about this condition. Disability also depends on a person's perception of her/his ability to perform activities associated with daily living. The United Nations (UN 2001) noted that disability rates from diverse national data sources are not yet comparable across the world because of differences in definitions, concepts, and methods. A major point in this chapter is that the two major designs for collecting data, census and survey, register disability differently, resulting in different numbers of people with disabilities.

Regional comparisons can be very misleading if the methodological differences are not taken into account. The use of different measurement instruments, the older age structure, as well as the larger capacity to observe and diagnose various kinds of disabilities in developed countries are likely factors for the higher rates of disability generally recorded in developed countries. In addition to the type of measurement instrument used, estimates of the proportion of disabled people in a population can also vary depending on whether disabled people are identified by using a 'disability screen' or an 'impairment screen'. African and Asian countries tend to use impairment screens in their censuses, surveys, and registration systems, and generally report lower rates than countries in Europe and North America, which tend (with some exceptions) to use disability screens. These sources can be used to examine the prevalence of disability, but they are not directly comparable because they use different approaches to estimating and measuring disability.

Prevalence of disability

There are relatively few censuses, surveys, and registration sources of information on disability in developing countries, and conceptual and definitional problems abound. However, several attempts have been made to find out roughly how many people in the world are disabled, what the main causes of disability are, and how the disabilities encountered in different countries and regions affect quality of life.

In 1981, the first estimates by the WHO were that 10 percent of any population was disabled (WHO 2011). Later, these figures were modified to 6 or 7 percent, giving a global figure of 245 million disabled people (Ingstad and Whyte 1995). The proportion of disabled people per national population varies between less than 1 percent in Peru and 21 percent in Austria, given differences in data collection designs, definitions, concepts, and methods (Elwan 1999). However in 1992, this estimate was modified to 4 percent for developing countries and 7 percent for industrialized countries. There is no consensus as to which figures to use. Reported disability prevalence rates from around the world vary dramatically, for example, from under 1 percent in Kenya and Bangladesh to 20 percent in New Zealand (Mont 2007a).

Does this mean that the number of disabled people in Bangladesh is 20 times higher than among people living in Kenya? Are these figures comparable? This is a serious issue to be considered by the researchers, policymakers and planners, and international organizations that work for people living with disabilities. This variation is caused by several factors: deciding a definition of disability, different methodologies of data collection, and variation in the quality of the study design. The result is that generating disability prevalence rates that are understandable and internationally comparable is a difficult enterprise. This situation is complicated further by the idea that there is no single correct definition of disability, that the nature and severity of disabilities vary greatly, and that how one measures disability differs depending on the purpose for measuring it. A higher estimated figure is sometimes used when learning disabilities are included.

The quality of information collected depends in large part on the validity and reliability of the questions. Designing a questionnaire is both an art and a science, and in the early stage of developing a questionnaire a number of issues must be considered, preferably in consultation with persons with disabilities. Using these individuals and their families to test and refine questions is an excellent pre-test approach (United Nations 2001). Thus, understanding the number of people with disabilities and their circumstances can improve efforts to remove disabling barriers and provide services to allow people with disabilities to participate. Collecting appropriate statistical and research data at the national and international levels has been a challenging issue in order to implement internationally agreed development goals for disabled people.

Measuring disability with the census method

The census is a country's most important data collection activity. The primary objective of a census is to count the population present or residing in the country and the absentee population living abroad. Generally, a national population census covers a range of information: age, sex, education, language, ethnicity, religion, occupation, income and assets, fertility, mortality, migration, and disability. A census format offers only limited space and time for questions on any one topic, including disability and human functioning. For countries that do not have regular, special population-based disability surveys or disability modules in ongoing surveys, the census can be the only information source on the frequency and distribution of disability and functioning in the population at the national, regional, and local level.

The World Health Survey, a face-to-face household survey in 2002–2004, is the largest multinational health and disability survey ever, using a single set of questions and consistent methods to collect comparable data across countries. In all countries, vulnerable groups, such as women, those in the poorest wealth quintile, and older people, had a higher prevalence of disability. For all these groups the rate was higher in developing countries. The prevalence of disability in lower-income countries among people aged 60 years and above, for instance, was 43.4 percent, compared with 29.5 percent in higher income countries (WHO and the World Bank 2011).

Reported disability prevalence rates with the census method vary widely (see Table 8.1). In many developed countries, the rates are quite high. The prevalence rates in the USA and Canada are 19.4 percent and 18.5 percent, respectively (Mont 2007a). Developing countries often report very low disability rates, for instance, below 1 percent in Kenya and Bangladesh. These rates vary for a number of reasons: different notions of disability, different measurement methodologies, and variation in the quality of measurement.

Different countries use different approaches to measure disability in their national census. Some countries include a specific question in the census questionnaire, for instance: *Do you or any member of the household have a disability?* This method generates the lowest rates of disability. The positive response rate to this question is typically in the 1–3 percent range. By using this method, the disability rate of Nigeria, Jordan, Philippines, Turkey, and Mauritania was found to be 0.5 percent, 1.2 percent, 1.3 percent, 1.4 percent, and 1.5 percent, respectively (Mont 2007a; WHO 2011).

Table 8.1 Prevalence of disability in different countries, using the census method

Country	Year	Percent of the population with a disability
The United States	2000	19.4
Canada	2001	18.5
Brazil	2000	14.5
The United Kingdom	1991	12.2
Poland	1988	10.0
Ethiopia	1984	3.8
Uganda	2001	3.5
Mali	1987	2.7
Mexico	2000	2.3
Chile	1992	2.2
India	2001	2.1
Colombia	1993	1.8
Bangladesh	1982	0.8
Kenya	1987	0.7

Source: Mont (2007a)

People in many societies may feel a social pressure to underreport disability. Respondents may not be enthusiastic to admit the presence of a person with disabilities in the household. One of the important issues to be taken into consideration is to design the census in such a way that the respondent will not perceive that they are asked about the stereotypes, often stigma, of disabilities. There are some limitations to use a census to collect data on disability, it being a condition that needs to be measured to consider several issues like intensity, duration, and framework. It is not a phenomenon that can be easily described with a simple classification between YES or NO. Questions that can cover various contexts, clarify terminology, and define multiple domains are required.

Some countries report higher rates of disability because they consider any condition that affects one's health, even those that do not necessarily have an impact on the range of activities a person could perform in daily life. This method asks if the person has some condition that affects a particular social role, such as attending school or being employed. For example, do you/does anyone in this household have a health problem or disability which prevents you/them from working or which limits the kind and amount of what you/they can do. By using this method, the disability rate of Poland, United Kingdom, Brazil, Canada, and the USA was found to be 10.0 percent, 12.2 percent, 14.5 percent, 18.5 percent, and 19.4 percent, respectively (Mont 2007a: 8).

The census data in developing countries focus on the individual's severe level of physical, mental, or emotional conditions. Such countries generally incorporate specific questions in their population census, such as the following:

- Does any member of your household have a physical, mental, or emotional condition that makes it difficult to do everyday jobs alone, such as visiting a doctor's office or shopping?
- Does any member of your household have a physical, mental, or emotional condition that seriously makes it difficult to concentrate, remember, or make decisions?
- Does anyone have difficulty with dressing or bathing?
- Does anyone have serious difficulty when walking or climbing stairs?
- Is anyone blind or does anyone have serious difficulty with seeing, even when wearing glasses?
- Is anyone deaf or does anyone have serious difficulty with hearing?

Countries that have a registration system providing regular data on persons with the most severe types of impairments may use census to complement these data on selected aspects of the broader concept of disability and functioning based on the ICF. Census data can be utilized for general planning programs and services (prevention and rehabilitation), monitoring selected aspects of disability trends, and evaluation of national programs and services concerning the equalization of opportunities in the country. However, for international comparison of selected aspects of disability prevalence in countries, one should be serious regarding its operational definition.

Compared to the more detailed and more numerous questions posed in surveys, the general census shows lower figures of prevalence of disability. For example, a common question in a census is this: *Is anyone in the household disabled?* This question generates lowest disability rates both in developed and developing countries. Another way of asking is this: *Does any member of this household have any difficulty in moving, seeing, hearing, speaking, or having learning problems?* Though the theme is the same, the way the question has been asked can provide higher rates of disability compared to the more simple way of asking the question.

The former way of formulating and asking questions to the household head or to the senior person in the household generates the lowest rates of disability, typically in the 1–3 percent range. Surveys among the same population using an approach that emphasizes functional ability yield estimates in the 10–20 percent range.

The reasons for not claiming oneself as a 'disabled person' are many. People may feel stigma or shame at identifying themselves as disabled. The question *Do you or any member of your family have a disability?* is inadequate to pick up mental and psychological disabilities, which tend to be particularly stigmatizing and are sometimes more easily hidden. Likewise, people who can walk slowly within their home and in the kitchen garden, but are incapable of walking more than one hour, may perceive their situation as not severe enough to consider oneself disabled. A person with a condition that affects a particular social role, such as attending school or being employed can be identified by asking, for example, *Do you/does anyone in this household have a health problem or disability which prevents you/them from working or which limits the kind or amount of work you/they can do?* If one calculates the prevalence rate of disability based on the response of this question, it certainly would be high.

It is also important to note that the concept of normal functioning varies across various cultures, age or even income groups. For example, elderly people with significant limitations and significant difficulties performing basic activities may not identify themselves as having a disability because, in their minds, the activity limitations are related to their age.

Measuring disability with the survey method

In general, surveys tend to report higher disability rates than censuses because they offer several dimensions in more extensive surveys. Short sets of disability questions that can be included in censuses, and extended sets suitable for surveys, are being developed and tested. In some surveys, the respondent is read a list of conditions, such as polio, epilepsy, paralysis, and others, and is asked if they have any of them. Mont (2007a) proposed several limitations to this approach. First, many people may not know their diagnosis, particularly when it comes to mental and psychological conditions. Second, knowledge about one's diagnosis is probably correlated with variables such as education, socio-economic status, and access to health services, thus introducing a potential bias in the collected data. And finally, the functional effects of a particular condition can vary widely. For example, untreated diabetes can lead to profound functional limitations such as blindness or the loss of limbs. Diabetes that is properly managed can have a relatively minor impact on someone's life. The same thing is true for something like the amputation of a leg. With proper medical treatment and a prosthetic, a person may have few limitations when it comes to daily life. Poor treatment, on the other hand, can lead to a series of painful and dangerous infections.

The disability status among the elderly is best assessed through questions of Activities of Daily Living (ADL), such as bathing, eating, moving, dressing, and toileting (UN 2001). The term ADL refers to a set of common, daily activities, the performance of which is required for personal self-care and independent living. ADLs are, therefore, a measure for the ability to perform, and ultimately of the quality of life associated with the functional status.

A person is classified as disabled if she/he has difficulty performing any ADLs. Questions that focus on basic activities or major body functions serve as better screens. In fact, a question such as *Do you have difficulty walking?* may pick up mobility limitations resulting not only from paralysis and amputation, but also serious heart problems or other medical conditions. A question such as *Do you have difficulty holding a conversation with others?* may pick up stuttering, loss of speech due to stroke, autism, or several other conditions. And for most purposes, it is the functional status that catches the attention, and how that impacts someone's life, and not necessarily the cause, medical or otherwise.

Of course, for a study designed to uncover the best approaches towards preventing disabilities, the cause and age of the onset could be important data. For example, there are two visually impaired persons, both 25 years old. One has been blind since birth and the other recently blinded in an accident. Although both have the same medical condition or impairment – blindness – they fall on very different parts of the functional continuum. The person who has never been able to see has spent his/her whole life accommodating to the world. This person will score lower on a functional scale than the recently blinded one. And as time goes by, the person who has only a short experience of living with blindness will surely cope with the new situation by learning new skills that meet new conditions, and hopefully begin to modify the environment to better suit relevant needs.

Instrumental Activities of Daily Living (IADL) is another approach similar to the ADLs, but with more demanding tasks. Examples include whether a person has problems managing money, shopping for groceries, or maintaining her/his household. The question to be asked are these: *Do you have any difficulty in moving, seeing, hearing, speaking, or learning, that has lasted, or is expected to last, six months or more?* This approach is also complicated if the desire is to have a measure that is internationally comparable. For example, 'bathing oneself' or 'dressing oneself' can have very different connotations in rural and urban situations, for the rich and the poor. Dressing in pants and a loose fitting shirt is different than dressing in something as complicated as a sari.

Thus, the prevalence of disability in surveys (see Table 8.2) in different countries varies across countries based on the disability framework of the state, legal, economic, and biomedical institutions as well as the concept of personhood, identity, and sense of being valued. The notions of citizenship, of compensations, and sense of value lost through

Table 8.2 Prevalence of disability in different countries, using the survey method

Country	Year	Percent of the population with a disability
New Zealand	1996	20.0
Australia	2000	20.0
Uruguay	1992	16.0
Spain	1986	15.0
Austria	1986	14.4
Zambia	2006	13.1
Sweden	1988	12.1
Ecuador	2005	12.1
The Netherlands	1986	11.6
Nicaragua	2003	10.3
Germany	1992	8.4
China	1987	5.0
Italy	1994	5.0
Egypt	1996	4.4

Source: Mont (2007a)

impairment and added through rehabilitation are institutionally rein-forced constituents of disability as a cultural construct. In developing countries where such institutional infrastructure exists only to a limited degree, reported disability is low (Ingstad and Whyte 1995). On the other hand, in many developed countries, people may also exaggerate disability at work in order to justify receiving disability benefits.

WHO (2008) has developed a 12-question set of Disability Assess-ment Schedule (WHODAS 2.0), including questions about difficul-ties with health related conditions, such as diseases or illnesses, other health problems that may be short or long lasting, injuries, mental or emotional problems, and problems with alcohol or drugs. Respon-dents are asked to think back over the last 30 days, trying to remem-ber how much difficulty she/he had doing the activities mentioned in Table 8.3. For each question, only one response is allowed.

Table 8.3 The WHO set of disability assessment

Level of difficulty	None	Mild	Moderate	Severe	Extreme	Unable
Standing for long periods, such as 30 minutes.						
Taking care of your household responsibilities.						
Learning a new task, for example, learning how to get to a new place.						
How much of a problem did you have joining in community activities (e.g. festivities, religious or other activities) in the same way as anyone else can?						
How much have you been emotionally affected by your health problems?						
Concentrating on doing something for ten minutes.						
Walking a long distance such as a kilometer (or equivalent).						
Washing your whole body.						
Difficulties getting dressed.						
Dealing with people you do not know.						

WHODAS 2.0 was developed through an international collaboration, with the aim of developing a single generic instrument for assessing health status and disability across different cultures and settings.

The WHO global burden of disease estimate

The first *Global Burden of Disease* study was commissioned in 1990 by the World Bank to assess the relative burden of premature mortality and disability from different diseases, injuries, and various risk factors. WHO reassessed the Global Burden of Disease for 2000–2004, drawing on available data to produce estimates of incidence, prevalence, severity, duration, and mortality for more than 130 health conditions in 17 sub-regions throughout the world. This report estimated that 15.3 percent of the world population had "moderate or severe disability," while 2.9 percent experienced "severe disability" (WHO and the World Bank 2011).

The Global Burden of Disease has given considerable attention to the internal consistency and comparability of estimates across the population for specific diseases and causes of injury, severity, and distributions of limitations in functioning. It is important, however, to note that national survey and census data cannot be compared directly with the World Health Survey or Global Burden of Disease estimates because there is no consistent approach across countries to disability definition and survey questions.

The disability situation in Nepal

Studies in Nepal have shown varying estimates of disabled persons. Censuses and surveys have taken different approaches to measure disability. They have covered only a few disability-relevant questions, and provided limited information about participation and activity difficulties. Surveys provide richer information through more comprehensive questions. Some surveys also provide information on the origin of impairments, the degree of assistance provided, service accessibility, and unmet needs.

The 1971 Census referred to persons in Nepal with disabilities as the 'economically inactive' population due to 'physical disability'. This definition included four types of disability: blindness, deafness, deaf-mute, or other physical impairments. The study indicated a national disability rate of 1.5 percent of the total population ten years or older (JICA 2002). The National Population Census of 1981, 1991, and 2001 (see Table 8.4) stated the disability rates as 0.5 percent, 1.5 percent, and 0.46 percent, respectively (CBS 1995, 2003).

The 2011 Nepal Population Census formulated a specific question related to disability: *What is the physical and mental disability of (Name)?* The options were the following: 1. Not disabled. 2. Physically disabled. 3. Blind and low vision. 4. Deaf and hard-of-hearing. 5. Deaf-blind. 6. Speech problem. 7. Mental illness. 8. Intellectually disabled. 9. Multiple disabled (see Table 8.5). The response given by the head of the household or by another person in the household was circled by the enumerator. The 2011 Population Census reported a 1.94 percent disability prevalence rate of the total population.

Is there data consistency among the various censuses? The answer is YES. In each census, the disabled population in Nepal is less than 2 percent. However, it is also argued that the census data focused exclusively on a narrow choice of impairments.

Table 8.4 Types of disability in the 2001 Population Census

Disability type	Number of people with disability	Percent of the total population
Physical	40,798	0.18
Blindness /Low Vision	16,526	0.07
Deaf /Hard to Hearing	25,540	0.11
Mentally Retarded	13,171	0.06
Multiple Disable	7,760	0.03
Total	103,795	0.46

Source: CBS (2003)

Table 8.5 Types of disability in the 2011 Population Census

Disability type	Number of people with disability	Percent of the total population
Physical	186,457	0.70
Blindness /Low Vision	94,765	0.36
Deaf /Hard to Hearing	79,307	0.30
Deaf-Blind	9,436	0.04
Speech Problem	58,855	0.22
Mental Disable	30,997	0.12
Intellectual Disable	14,888	0.06
Multiple Disable	38,616	0.15
Total	513,321	1.94

Source: CBS (2012)

High disability prevalence tends to have been based on data collected through surveys that record activity limitations and participation restriction, in addition to impairments. The underlying purpose of the survey, whether a disability-specific program intervention or a general survey, also affects how people respond.

The disability sample survey of 1980 reported a prevalence of about 3 percent disability among the total population. This study defined "persons with disabilities as those who by virtue of congenital disease, acquired disease, or injury, are incapable of living an independent personal or social life, or engaging in gainful employment, or acquiring normal education consistent with his/her age or sex" (JICA 2002).

A study carried out in five districts in 1991 stated that 16.6 percent of children aged over five were deaf. The Mother and Infant Research Activities (MIRA) conducted a study focusing on the 'Prevalence of Childhood and Adolescents Disabilities in the Makawanpur district' (Sauvey et al. 2005). The data were collected in all households in 24 VDCs in the Makawanpur district, from September 1999 to June 2000. The study aimed to determine the number of children and young people reported by family members to have a disability, and to classify impairments leading to disability. Each head of the household (or, if not present, the next more senior person) was invited to respond to a questionnaire including two questions about disability: (1) *Is there anyone in your household under the age of 20 who has a disability?* (2) If yes, *What is the nature of the disability?* People under the age of 20 with a disability lived in 733 of 28,376 households, a household prevalence of 2.58 percent. A total of 829 people under the age of 20 were reported as having a disability, that is 0.95 percent of the population (Sauvey et al. 2005).

A Danish International Development Agency (DANIDA) funded study estimated the disability prevalence rate in Nepal as 5.04 percent (DANIDA 1995). Another study, also funded by DANIDA, covered eight districts. This study classified disabilities into five categories (hearing, visual, physical, mental, and intellectual), and indicated a prevalence of 4.55 percent (CERID et al. 1995). In 2005, the BP Koirala Institute of Health Sciences (BPKIHS) conducted a disability survey in the Sunsari district. Among a total of 640,259 individuals, 31,160 individuals (4.87 percent) were disabled, being 6.89 percent of the households (Karki et al. 2008).

A national survey on 'Situation Analysis of Disability in Nepal' was carried out in 1999–2000, under the aegis of the National Planning Commission and the Social Welfare Council, funded by UNICEF. The main purpose of the study was to develop a comprehensive definition of all kinds of disabilities and to obtain nation-wide data and information about the situation and services for persons with disabilities in Nepal. The definition considered a person to be disabled if the person could not perform the daily activities of life considered normal for a human being within the specified age group, and where the person needed special care, support, and some sort of rehabilitation services (National Planning Commission et al. 2001).

The study was conducted in 30 districts spread over the country's 15 eco-development regions. A sample of 13,005 households, covering a population of 75,944, was included in the study. Based on the definition adopted for the study, the prevalence of disability was estimated to be 1.63 percent of the total population, with estimates of 1.65 percent in rural areas and 1.43 percent in urban areas (National Planning Commission et al. 2001). Similarly, in 2006, WATCH, a nongovernmental organization based in Kathmandu, carried out a survey in three geographic areas of Nepal, covering a total of 19,210 persons in 3,397 households. A total of 355 persons with disabilities were identified, giving an overall disability prevalence of 1.84 percent (Shrestha et al. 2009). These survey findings are closer to the findings of the national censuses in Nepal.

The discrepancies between the estimates of disabilities in Nepal could be due to a lack of a standard definition of disability (National Federation of Disabled-Nepal 2010). Therefore, there is a need to clearly spell out the definition of disability for Nepal and then investigate the prevalence of disability.

Conclusion

The heterogeneity of the conceptual framework and insufficient recognition of the importance of indicator accuracy, the age factor, and the socio-economic characteristics of the population under study all affect the prevalence disability rate in any country or place. Although census data are quite detailed, disability is not a phenomenon that can be easily categorized with a simple binary classification. Thus, census data can underestimate some forms of disability. People may not report certain socially stigmatized conditions, such as alcohol and drug-related conditions, and mentally related problems.

On the other hand, in the focused surveys, disability data can be too inclusive and measure minor difficulties in functioning that do not require assistance from another person, group, or any support from a state agency. This method also has the potential to count people with disabilities more than once. It is difficult to ascertain whether the increase in disability rates is real or a statistical anomaly resulting from methodological and conceptual problems. For example, a greater willingness by people to reply, when interviewed in surveys, that they have a disability, may be the result of economic incentives to report disability in order to benefit from disability support programs, or be the result of a greater acceptance of, and openness to, people with disabilities in the society. The prevalence can also be affected by the number and types of questions, the scale indicating the levels of difficulty, the range of explicit disabilities, and the methodology used. The different disability rates obtained in census and survey methods are mainly due to the domain included and the threshold for defining a disability.

The variations across countries as shown, for example, in Table 8.1 and Table 8.2, can be more reliable when the questions become more specific and are used in a similar way. In practice, disability should be appropriately measured according to the purpose for which it will be used. A collaboration and coordination between various initiatives to measure disability prevalence at the global, regional, and national levels is urgent. WHO, an umbrella organization, can be a key facilitator to solve methodological debates and issues.

Furthermore, a dedicated disability survey should be carried out to gain extensive information on disability and activity limitations, health conditions associated with disability, and the use of, and need for, services. Such information allows researchers and policymakers to understand disability, instigating prevention programs, and modifying interventions is a cross-sector matter.

Note

1 A version of this chapter originally appeared as 'Challenges to Measure and Compare Disability: A Methodological Concern', *Dhaulagiri Journal of Sociology and Anthropology*, 6: 1–24, 2012. Used with permission.

References

CBS. 1995. *Population Monograph of Nepal*. Kathmandu: CBS.

CBS. 2003. *Population Monograph of Nepal*, Vol. 1. Kathmandu: CBS.

CBS. 2012. *Nepal Population and Housing Census 2011*. Kathmandu: CBS.

CERID, SED, BPEP and DANIDA. 1995. *Disabled People of Nepal*. Tribhuvan University Research Centre for Educational Innovation and Development; Basic and Primary Education Program. Kathmandu: Danish International Development Agency.

DANIDA. 1995. *Disability Survey of Kanchanpur District*. Kathmandu: Danish International Development Agency.

Ellis, Katie and Mike Kent. 2011. *Disability and New Media*. New York: Routledge.

Elwan, Ann. 1999. *Poverty and Disability: A Survey of Literature*. Washington, DC: The World Bank.

Hutchison, Tom. 1995. "The Classification of Disability." *Archives of Disease in Childhood* 73: 91–99.

Ingstad, Benedicte and Susan Reynolds Whyte. 1995. "Disability and Culture: An Overview." In Benedicte Ingstad and Susan Reynolds Whyte, eds., *Disability and Culture*, pp. 3–32. Berkeley: University of California Press.

JICA. 2002. *Country Profile on Disability: Kingdom of Nepal*. Kathmandu: JICA.

Karki, R., B. K. Yadav, A. Chakravartty and D. B. Shrestha. 2008. "The Prevalence and Characteristics of Disability in Eastern Nepal." *Kathmandu University Medical Journal* 6(21): 94–97.

Mont, Daniel. 2007a. *Measuring Disability Prevalence*. Washington, DC: The World Bank.

Mont, Daniel. 2007b. "Measuring Health and Disability." *Lancet* 369: 1658–1663.

National Federation of Disabled-Nepal. 2010. *Baseline Survey of Persons with Disability of Having Disability ID Card*. Kathmandu: National Federation of Disabled Nepal.

National Planning Commission, UNICEF, and New ERA. 2001. *A Situation Analysis of Disability in Nepal*. Kathmandu: National Planning Commission, UNICEF, New ERA.

Sauvey, S., D. Osrin, D. S. Manandhar, A. M. Costello and S. Wirz. 2005. "Prevalence of Childhood and Adolescent Disabilities in Rural Nepal." *Indian Pediatrics* 42(17): 697–702.

Shrestha, Sarmila, Narayan Kaji Shrestha and Sunil Deepak. 2009. "A Community Assessment of Poverty and Disability among Specific Rural Population Groups in Nepal." *Asia Pacific Disability Rehabilitation Journal* 20(1): 83–98.

UN-ESCAP. 2010. *Disability at Glance 2010: A Profile of 36 Countries and Areas in Asia and the Pacific*. Bangkok: Economic and Social Commission for Asia and Pacific Social Development Division, United Nations.

United Nations. 2001. *Guidelines and Principles for the Development of Disability Statistics*. New York: United Nations.

WHO. 1976. *Document A29/INFDOCI*. Geneva: WHO.

WHO. 1980. *International Classification of Impairment, Disabilities and Handicaps: A Manual of Classification Relating to the Consequences of Disease*. Geneva: WHO.

WHO. 2002. *International Classification of Functioning, Disability and Health (ICF)*. Geneva: WHO.

WHO. 2004. *Global Burden of Disease Report*. Geneva: WHO.

WHO. 2008. *WHODAS 2.0*. Geneva: WHO.

WHO and the World Bank. 2011. *World Report on Disability*. Geneva: WHO.

9 Trade in health service

Unfair competition of pharmaceutical products in Nepal[1]

Pharmaceuticals are playing an important role in people's life. Social, behavioral, or bodily conditions are treated or deemed by doctors to be in need of treatment with medical drugs. Growing pharmaceuticalization reflects progress in the medical sciences, and people get medications for illnesses that were previously undiagnosed or untreated. Pharmaceuticalization is also driven by industry promotion and advertising of specific drug products to the medical profession (Abraham 2010).

Pharmaceuticals are indispensable in any health system; by complementing other types of health care services they can reduce mortality and morbidity rates and enhance the quality of life. Therefore, access to health care and essential medicines is increasingly being viewed as a fundamental human right (WHO 2009). Yet the abilities of pharmaceuticals to save lives, reduce suffering, and improve health depends on these being of good quality, safe, available, affordable, and proper use. It is estimated that one third of the global population do not have regular access to essential medicine. Furthermore, one third of the developing countries either have no regulatory authority or only limited capacity to regulate the medicine market (WHO 2009). The pharmaceutical sector is highly vulnerable to corruption and unethical practices (WHO 2006, 2009), due in part to the high market value of pharmaceutical products. Moreover, the stakeholders involved are numerous, diverse, and have different objectives. They include manufacturers, wholesalers, retailers, prescribers, sales representatives, regulators, policymakers, and researchers.

The pharmaceutical industry applies a large proportion of its resources to marketing and advertizing operations (Petryna and Kleinman 2006). One central issue in the debate about the pharmaceutical industry has been whether it is primarily driven by innovation or marketing. Information about the pharmaceutical companies' promotional expenditures is rarely available and is questioned by the public health experts and consumer rights activists. A majority of critics of the pharmaceutical policy in the developing countries seem to favor a drastic regulation of health services, including the pharmaceuticals (Van der Geest 1984). Their basic idea is that the profit maximization by definition is pathogenic because it puts profit before people. The structure of relations between manufacturers and the supply chain (the importer, wholesaler, and retailer), between manufacturer and prescriber, involves something more like reciprocal access to guarded resources (Lakoff 2006). Prescription drug promotion practices that involve giving financial grants and valuable items to doctors and retailers are common in Nepal (Subedi 2001; GPAN 2007; Thapa 2007a).

Although the history of drug manufacturing in Nepal dates back to 1968, when experimental production started at the Royal Drug Research Laboratory (now Nepal Drug Limited), the growth in the public and private pharmaceutical industry was slow. The pharmaceutical industry in Nepal developed rapidly after the introduction of a neo-liberal economic policy during the 1980s.

Nepal's pharmaceutical market is dominated with Indian products, but the domestic manufacturers are increasing their market share. The Nepali market size for pharmaceutical products is not big compared to the market of the neighboring countries. The consciousness about quality products in the pharmaceutical sector is growing by consumers as well as by producers.

On July 17, 2007, the Government of Nepal's Department of Drug Administration (DDA) released its Guidelines on Ethical Promotion of Medicine. The objective was to enhance ethical promotion of medicine to support and encourage the improvement of health care through the rational use of medicine and to discourage unethical practices. The guideline focused some of the key issues. First, all informational and persuasive activities by the manufacturers and distributors should take place only with respect to medicine legally available in the country. Promotion should be in keeping with the National Drug Policy and in compliance with the Drug Act and regulations. Second, prescriptive drugs should never be advertised in any form of printing or electronic media targeting the general public. Third, pharmaceutical industries should develop a manual on the promotion of medicine to ensure full compliance with the guidelines and to review and monitor all of their promotional activities and materials. Fourth, manufacturers and distributors should have a policy not to provide any kind of inducement in cash or kind, including, but not limited to, free medicines to prescribers, dispensers, or retail pharmacies as a promotional practice.

Fifth, medical representatives must display the highest professional and ethical standards at all times. Under no circumstance should medical representatives pay a fee in order to gain access to health care practitioners. They should not offer inducements to prescribers and the dispensers, and the main part of the medical representatives' remuneration should not be directly related to the volume of the sales they generate. Sixth, the foreign companies importing their products to Nepal should either open their office in Nepal or that the importer would be responsible on their behalf.

The guidelines, however, could not properly be implemented due to the conflict of interests among various stakeholders. In a complex system such as the pharmaceutical trade, the many vested interests and players that blame other groups do not reflect critically upon their own practice (Harper and Jeffery 2009). This chapter describes the historical context of the ethical guidelines and the interests of various stakeholders, focusing particularly on the issue of bonuses or gifts. This is not only interesting for producers, distributors, and retailers, but also one of the state's and the general public's major concerns.

Methods and materials

When the DDA released its Guidelines on Ethical Promotion of Medicine in 2007, the Nepal Chemist and Druggists Association (NCDA), one of the major stakeholders supposed to follow the Guidelines, forwarded a 12-point demand to the concerned authority to nullify the guidelines. Though NCDA is a non-governmental organization, it represents the interests of the importers, wholesalers, and retailers. On August 6, 2007, NCDA announced that it would stop importing drugs from the very next day, as part of its protest. This sensitized the issue in the public sphere.

To explore the ongoing discourse and the conflicting interests, several stakeholders were studied during the implementation of the guidelines. Documents and papers were reviewed, and a series of formal and informal interactions were initiated with the key stakeholders like the Association of Pharmaceuticals Producers of Nepal (APPON), the Nepal Medical Council (NMC), the Nepal Pharmaceutical Association (NPA), the Graduate Pharmacists' Association, Nepal (GPAN), the NCDA, the Nepal Medical Association (NMA), the Nepal Pharmacy Council (NPC), the Nepal Medical and Sales Representative Association (NMSRA), and the DDA. A total of 21 representatives of all these organizations were interviewed once or several times, depending upon their response with other stakeholders. The interviews were conducted in October–December 2007. The interviews were conducted in Nepali, and then transcribed into English. The rest of this chapter presents the results from these interviews.

Results and discussion

The chapter starts with a description of the contexts of the guidelines and explores the discourse of various organizations involved during the formulation of ideas, preparations of the draft report, and the challenges faced during the implementation of the guidelines.

The international context

The governance of pharmaceutical production and consumption is a dynamic interplay between a number of different stakeholders, their positions, interests, and commitments. A range of professional groups locates themselves around knowledge and expertise in a pharmaceutical chain. The transnational pharmaceutical companies have interests both as commercial players and as bodies with public responsibility for combating disease and improving the population's health status.

Between the late 1920s and the mid-1970s, all western industrialized countries introduced government regulations of drug safety and efficacy, as well as quality. The timing of such regulations varied from 1928 in Norway, 1935 in Sweden, 1962 in the USA, and 1971 in the UK (Abraham 2008). The rationale for the historical emergence of pharmaceutical regulations was the consciousness about the pharmaceuticals and of unethical drug promotion by companies, and to provide access to information about drug risks and benefits.

Following the WHO conference on the rational use of drugs, held in Nairobi in November 1985, WHO prepared a revised drug strategy that was endorsed by the 33rd World Health Assembly in May 1986. This strategy included, among several components, the establishment of ethical criteria for drug promotion based on the updating and extension of the ethical and scientific criteria established in 1968 by the 21st World Health Assembly. The criteria were prepared on the basis of a draft elaborated by an international group of experts. The main objective for developing ethical criteria for medical drug promotion was to support and encourage the improvement of health care through the rational use of medical drugs.

These criteria constitute general principles for ethical standards that the government could adapt to national conditions appropriate to their political, economic, cultural, social, educational, scientific and technical situation, laws and regulations, disease profile, therapeutic traditions, and the level of development of their health system (Raut 2008). They apply to prescription and non-prescription medical drugs ('over-the-counter drugs'), and also generally to appropriate traditional medicines and to any other product promoted as medicine. It was also clearly stated that the criteria could be used by people working in various fields: government administration; the pharmaceutical industry (manufacturers and distributors); the promotion industry (advertising agencies, market research organizations, etc.); health personnel involved in the prescription, dispensing, supply, and distribution of drugs; universities and other teaching institutions; professional associations; patients and consumer groups; and the professional and general media (including publishers and editors of medical journals and related publications).

All these actors were encouraged to use the criteria appropriately to their spheres of competence, activity, and responsibility. They also were encouraged to take the criteria into account when developing their own sets of ethical standards related to drug promotion. It was stated that the criteria did not constitute legal obligations, but that governments might adopt legislation or other measures based on them as they deemed fit. The WHO ethical criteria cover a wide range of promotional activities like advertising, medical representatives, samples, symposia and scientific meetings, and post-marketing scientific studies.

The national context

The gate for allopathic medicine in Nepal opened only after the British Residency, established in Kathmandu in 1816, built a small hospital for the residency staff. This hospital also provided services to local people. The number of hospitals in Nepal gradually increased after the establishment of the Bir Hospital in 1890.

The distribution of imported medicines in Nepal started much earlier than the first attempts in the 1950s to manufacture allopathic medicine in Nepal. The expansion of the country's market brought by the construction of the east–west highway and other link roads, paved the way for the pharmaceutical companies to reach a wider market.

The idea of producing allopathic medicine in Nepal developed only after the 1955 master plan for using medicinal plants was implemented in 1961. As per the plan, the Royal Drug Research Laboratory (RDRL) was established in 1964, which, along with various research activities, started manufacturing allopathic medicine in 1968.

The Drug Act of 1978 was promulgated in Nepal to prohibit the misuse or abuse of pharmaceutical materials as well as the false or misleading information relating to the efficacy and use of drugs, and to regulate and control the production, marketing, distribution, export–import, and storage and utilization of drugs which were not safe for people to use, not being efficacious or of standard quality. In 1986, eight years after the Drug Act was passed, the Government of Nepal published the National List of Essential Drugs based on the country's disease pattern as well as the relative merit of selected drugs in terms of cost, safety, and efficacy. This step also was taken in response to WHO's request to all member countries to have a list of essential drugs as per the country's need. This list was revised in 1992, 1997, and 2002, respectively. In accordance with the objectives of the 1991 National Health Policy, the National Drug Policy was implemented in 1995.

The Standards for Pharmaceutical Regulation and Care was implemented in 2002. It included indicators for monitoring and measuring good performance and to ensure quality service to meet people's needs. The document adapted the WHO/SEARO framework for developing health care standards and focused particularly on quality characteristics for drug regulatory control, drug supply and management, rational drug use, and safe disposal. This framework highlighted the principles for regularly controlling pharmaceutical sales promotion and advertisement by measuring the level of promotional activities, and to prevent and monitor perverse incentives for prescribers and dispensers.

By the end of July 2015, there were 60 allopathic medicine manufacturing and repacking companies, 27 of them being WHO-GMP certified. The pharmaceutical market has ample opportunity in Nepal with a current market share of approximately 40–45 percent.

The context of ethical guideline

Nepal being a small market with prospects for good possibilities for domestic pharmaceutical production, replacing imports has resulted in the development of industries. Bonuses and special incentives have played a major role in the promotional practices. This also has resulted in some unethical practices by most of the companies, including Indian ones. At this juncture, in 2006, the DDA proposed a study of the current promotional practices of the pharmaceutical companies in Nepal, a study that was supported by WHO. The study's main objective was to identify the current promotional practices of pharmaceutical products available in Nepal, and to assess the existing practices in context of the WHO criteria for drug promotion and its compliance with ethical promotion.

In 2005, the GPAN, in collaboration with the DDA and WHO, conducted a study on promotional practices in Nepal's pharmaceutical market. A total of 30 pharmaceutical companies were selected, 15 domestic and 15 Indian. The findings were presented during a seminar on February 3, 2007. The study revealed a wide variation in bonus schemes offered by the companies. For example, products for cardiac problems did not have bonus. Products like Amoxycillin and Ciprofloxacin were in the market with a bonus offer ranging from 10 percent to 100 percent. Albendazole 400 mg was another product with a bonus ranging from 20 percent to 100 percent. Vitamin B complexes had a 60 percent bonus offer, especially for 200 ml packs. The 100 ml packs were sold at a bonus offer half to that offered for 200 ml packs. Even products such as cough formula, anti ORS, were having a bonus system. The most commonly used bonus by every company was 10 percent and 70–100 percent as exceptional cases for certain products. However, some companies had been practicing a no-offer system for selling some selected products.

The study did not find any relationship between the WHO Good Manufacturing Practice (GMP) certified companies and a bonus offer. The bonus offer was practiced equally by the WHO–GMP certified companies, and by other companies. Some WHO–GMP certified companies even have offered good gift items such as TV to the prescribers. However, for certain products, some of the WHO–GMP certified companies had a maximum bonus offer of 20 percent without any extra benefit offer. The gift items being offered were carpets, pens, blankets, bed sheets, iron, calculator, TV, etc. The companies also had practiced offering a bonus for products that the DDA had already decided an unethical practice.

The companies had gone beyond ethical norms to provide a special incentive of personal benefit from the sale of products in quantity, while forgetting the issues of quality and patient benefits. It was very clear that the retailers benefitted from maximum bonus offers and long-term limits on credit. The study highlighted that the retailers' substitution of prescription with products with a higher offer, had resulted in some setbacks regarding turnover growth for some companies that focused their promotion on an ethical prescription base.

Based on the research findings, the concerned stakeholders clearly felt the need for implementing guidelines on the ethical promotion of medicine in Nepal. The Guidelines on the Ethical Promotion of

Medicine was drafted and discussed with various stakeholders like APPON, NMC, NPA, GPAN, NCDA, NMA, NPC, and NMSRA, and the DDA implemented them from July 17, 2007. Although the term 'promotion' refers to all informational and persuasive activities by manufacturers and distributors, the effect of which is to induce the prescription, supply, purchase, and/or use of medicine, the DDA authority stated that the commonly used unethical practice is to provide expensive gifts, either in the form of cash or kind to the prescriber, sponsoring pleasure trips abroad, and in form of free medicine to the retailers.

Conflict of interest: one issue, many voices

Many stakeholders welcomed the Ethical Guidelines and argued that this policy would have a long-term beneficial effect for the nation and its people towards making a stronger and self-reliant Nepal. The former President of APPON admitted the unethical practices of medicine in Nepal:

> Of course, the unhealthy practices are rampant in the country while selling and marketing drugs [. . .]. There is a glaring trend to offer free goods and bonuses to the retailers. Comparing with the neighboring India, this sort of trend is more prevalent in Nepal. Only a certain number of companies are reaping undue advantages at the cost of the entire health sector of the country. This is also sure to hamper the ethical expansion of pharmaceutical companies. Nepali pharmaceutical companies are offering more commission to retailers than Indian companies of the same nature. The strategy adopted by the domestic pharmaceutical companies is gravitated towards the promotion of domestically manufactured drugs.
>
> (Vaidya 2008: 4)

He also acknowledged that pharmaceutical companies tended to bribe doctors to prescribe their medicines. He felt that without visionary interactions among all the stakeholders engaged in the pharmaceutical sector, the sector could not expect a dynamic development. The President of APPON admitted (Shrestha 2008: 64):

> Ideally, a code of conduct should come from within and it should not be imposed by any agencies. In the absence of any such activity from the private sector, the Government of Nepal took lead in

this matter and held rounds of discussions with all stakeholders before actually implementing the ethical guideline on pharmaceutical marketing. The problem started when the major stakeholders backed out and openly defied the government decision. This led to a chaotic situation in the pharmaceutical market.

During my informal dialogue with the manufacturers in 2007, most of the APPON members mentioned that individual manufacturers should be more responsible for a better implementation of the guidelines. The retailers related to the medicine trade are entitled to 16 percent, and wholesalers are entitled to a commission about 5–6 percent as per the provisions fixed by the Government of Nepal. The DDA and APPON reached an agreement to offer extra 10 percent commission on prescribed drugs and 20 percent on non-prescribed drugs to concerned retailers. So, why having a system that gave the dispenser an extra incentive in the form of discount or free medicine, which could be sold? This was a lucrative offer to the retailers for substituting the prescription (Thapa 2007b).

The NCDA, a key player in the distribution of drugs, voiced its reservation. Members of the NCDA argued that a handful of people, including the DDA, were trying to denigrate the reputation of the NCDA by putting the issue of a deal bonus in a bad light. They argued that the Ethical Guidelines suggested to drop the deal bonus. However, just dropping this option or enforcing the Ethical Guidelines, one could not be sure that the deal bonus scheme would be halted, and not resulting in drug prices going down. They argued that the profit would be transmitted straight to the producers, not to the people in general. They had seen that the DDA and APPON had conspired to victimize the retailers and argued that such regulation could be implemented unilaterally against NCDA. However, such actions required more discussions.

The NCDA also forwarded a 12-point demand as a prerequisite before the guidelines could be implemented. Most of the demands presented were not related to the guidelines. This action by the NCDA was in fact a strategy to cloud the bonus issue for the consumer. The NCDA even circulated a notice to its members (retailers and distributors), stating that they would refrain from importing, distributing, and selling drugs if the government did not look into their demands. A memorandum to this effect was given to the Health Secretary and the Health Minister. This resulted in a meeting between the NCDA and the Health Ministry officials, whereby the Ministry agreed to look into their demands in a positive light. However, this action on the part of the NCDA should be seen as another stumbling block because it distorted the context and delayed the implementation of the guidelines. A leading consumer activist contended that the Health Ministry's agreement was beyond its jurisdiction. He affirmed that the Minister's decision, by giving in to the pressure put forth by NCDA, went against the authority of the DDA's Drugs Decision Committee (DDC), and that such an action implied policy corruption.

During my interaction with Executive Committee members of NCDA, they repeatedly expressed a concern for the country's health situation and also about some issues in the Guidelines. Some members also argued that the Guidelines were very sophisticated and, therefore, could be implemented only in advanced countries like the USA, the UK, and Japan. When further asked about how to improve the situation, the simple answer was to have a less corrupted medical sector that would focus more on serving people.

The DDA chief's view was that a written code of ethics was required to obtain uniform behavior (Thapa 2007b). The DDA's leadership thought that the document should have been made by the companies, and that it was not something the government needed to do. In Nepal, none of the companies took the initiative to make such a document, and there were a lot of anomalies in the market after the government adopted a liberal policy for the pharmaceutical industry. As a result, the government had not paid much attention to the prices of medicine.

Despite its professional demand and some reservations regarding the guidelines, the NMSRA was quite positive towards the Ethical Guidelines. For instance, during the interview with the President of NMSRA, he said:

> The positive point of the ethical guidelines is that the foreign companies exporting their products to Nepal should either open their office in Nepal or the importer is made responsible on their behalf. It is also mentioned that the name of the marketing chief of domestic as well as foreign companies must be provided to the DDA and any change of person should be notified as soon as possible. If DDA implements this properly along with the registration of medical representatives, 60 percent of the ethical concern will be solved. For the remaining 40 percent, concerns are related to the behaviors of the prescribers and the retailers.

The President mentioned that the benefits and salaries of the medical representatives were determined based on the sales volume of the drugs of the particular company. In order to increase the sales volume of a specific company, their representatives used to go to wholesalers and the retailers who were under undue pressure from Indian companies to meet their targets. Also, doctors were increasingly demanding more and more elaborate gifts before they acted in ways that would enable the company representatives to meet their targets (Harper and Jeffery 2009). The President of NMSRA further said:

> In order to avoid over-promotion, the main part of the remuneration of the medical representatives should not directly be related to the volume of the sales. But in practices, this has been happening in Nepal. Most of the medical representatives should fulfill their quota. If we are able to sell our product above the quota provided, we get some kind of reward. If we are unable to fulfill the given quota, our job is at risk. If such situations continue, the ethical promotion of medicine becomes like a dream.

Members of the NMSRA thought that the implementation of the guidelines would help to reduce the price of medicine, benefitting people directly. If the bonus system was removed, only the manufacturers would benefit. "APPON seems positive towards the Ethical Guidelines because manufacturers want to cut down the bonus, but they don't want to change their prices, which is unfair and unethical," said the NMSRA Central Committee member.

The NMSRA's concern seems to be about the price of medicine. The NMSRA members told that the bonus varied from one company to another, one brand to another, one category to another. For the Indian companies, the bonus generally was about 20 percent for OTC drugs, and 10 percent for Antibiotics. They hardly gave bonus for lifesaving drugs. They did not see such consistency among the Nepali companies.

The Nepal Medical Council's views were straightforward. The former Registrar of the NMC mentioned that some doctors might have a very good relationship with specific companies, brands, and products. They might trust one specific company based on their own experience and not because of gifts and other benefits. Other people could say that Dr X is getting an advantage from the company Y so that he/she prescribed a specific brand. This might not be true. The former Registrar said:

> DDA is the main responsible body for the quality control but it has its own limitations. Inadequate human resources, incompetent human resources, lack of the support from other stakeholders, and lack of commitment of the people who are responsible for the

various activities, are some of the limiting factors of DDA. Likewise, APPON should monitor the fair business within the companies. One of the important points is that we are still depending upon the Indian companies and multinational companies, they have their business policy and we have not been able to enforce them for the ethical promotion of pharmaceutical products. We even do not know their promotional strategies.

Members of the NMC believed that the objective of the ethical guidelines would be to promote the rational use of medicine, discourage unethical practices, and to promote a healthy business among producers by not compromising the quality of medicine. The NMC's opinion was that after developing clear-cut guidelines and implementing them properly, it would be possible to put moral pressure on the Indian and multinational companies.

Another stakeholder, the NMA, fully supported the DDA's move to ensure ethical practice in the country's medical sector. Responding to the rumor that doctors demanded gifts and other benefits from the companies to prescribe their brands, the President of NMA said:

> The accusation that a majority of the doctors unethically take bribes from some pharmaceutical companies to prescribe their drugs does not hold any ground. While entering into the profession, the doctors take an oath to perform their duties with humanity, compassion, and dedication to the welfare of the sick people according to the best of their ability and judgment. To promote their brand, medical representatives provide samples of medicine to the doctors, which is not unethical. Some companies give calendars, pens, diaries to the doctors. This has been very common these days. This is not a secret and is widely acceptable all over the world.

He mentioned that the main players of the guidelines are the manufacturers and the retailers. If the ethical guidelines were implemented, the price of the medicine would certainly decrease. He further said:

> Doctors are not demanding any gifts, retailers are not demanding any gifts, but the manufacturers are pushing their drugs by giving gifts to the doctors and bonus to the retailers. This should be stopped as soon as possible. It has been very urgent to develop prescription substitution control mechanism, particularly in prescription substitution prone areas like major hospitals.

The NMA, however, accepted that pharmaceutical companies provided a small support for workshops and doctors' professional meetings. This did not mean that the doctors were supposed to prescribe, recommend, or promote their brands.

Price, substitution, and consumer health

Despite the numerous positive aspects of the guidelines, only the issue of 'bonus' has taken center stage in the debate. The bonus issue can also be linked to the prices of medicines and accompanying practices associated with the sales of medicines to the consumers. It is difficult for a person to know the reasonable price of a medicine. The price for the very same medicine, but of different brands, is often different. There are various factors influencing the prices, but the variation should be within a tolerable limit (Thapa 2007a). It is obvious that if the bonus is cut, also the price of the medicine should be cut, to the benefit of the buyers, that is the people.

The tremendous variation in the prices of medicines may affect the trust in the quality of medicine. Sometimes a price increase is due to unreasonable expenses on market promotion. Commenting on the scenario of drugs distribution and sales in Nepal, the General Secretary of Consumer Rights argued that bonuses, gifts to doctors, and expenses rendered for travel and seminar to doctors are rife, and are ultimately borne by the consumer. Citing an example from the Pokhara Zonal Hospital that had rented out space to a private pharmacy for one million rupees, the General Secretary claimed that the law categorically stated that each hospital had to run its own pharmacy. Furthermore, by pointing to irregularities in the drug distribution and sales regime, drug pricing, fake drugs, and lack of monitoring by the government, the General Secretary argued that the government's decision of August 2007 compounded the already deteriorating system of drug distribution and sales in Nepal.

Regarding the issue of retailers getting bonuses, some argued that the consumer should ask for a discount when purchasing medicine. It is better to provide a reasonable price rather than creating a situation where a consumer can ask for a discount. Quality medicine at reasonable prices should be the motto for all pharmaceutical industries (Thapa 2007a). Some unethical trends in the promotion of medicine have not only increased concern among the consumers, but also among the producers. As many products from various producers are exactly the same, the easiest way of promotion is persuasive action targeting the prescribers and/or the drug retailers. The pharmaceutical companies' practice of substituting medicines that are sold to the consumers is rife, and the issue of bonus directly impinges on this practice. This has also led to the market for pharmaceuticals to be promoted unethically. Lucrative offers to the prescriber may insist over prescription of medicine. Likewise, provision of various offers to retailer may encourage prescription substitution and dispensing medicine without prescription.

After the DDA introduced the guidelines, it also made an effort to reduce the price of some medicines, and published them in the Gorkhapatra National Daily. People were expecting a cut in the price of medicine, at least from Nepali manufacturers, but it did not happen.

Challenges to implement the guidelines

The Guidelines do not have any legal status, so practice is voluntary; one can either abide by them or not abide at all. There is still confusion regarding the importers. Thus, the guidelines' status as of now is that their effect is very limited and that Nepal has to wait a few years to see the results of the guidelines. The DDA discussed possible solutions and also tried to call for one or two meetings to thrash out what needed to be changed.

The Government of Nepal tried to revise the Guidelines and make them a mandatory Act. Almost all stakeholders agreed that all the margins should be transparent, for the wholesalers as well as the retailers, and there should not be any under-the-table activities. Hence to regulate ethical marketing, also the regulators must improve their capacity, training, and expertise to act on complaints from the public, voluntary organizations, and from the pharmaceutical industry itself. Internal training, promotional practices, and post-market surveillance systems within pharmaceutical companies must be subjected to regulatory audit. However, these stakeholders have not shown keen interest to work together for the pharmaceutical governance in Nepal.

The guidelines are almost entirely concerned with the macrostructures of drug distribution; the actual users of pharmaceuticals hardly come into the picture (Van der Geest 1984). Sometimes, a rational drug policy may not always be to the advantage of the policymaking elites in Nepal. Consumer groups who know about people's health conditions and economic situation could play an important role in exploring the options for consumer action. Social scientists can add important information in this respect.

Conclusion

An effective functioning of the pharmaceutical system is dependent on the transparency of the process, and ability to hold individuals, organizations, agencies, and companies accountable for adhering to standard procedures, norms, laws, and regulations. When the medicines are prescribed and dispensed more for the financial interests of the prescribers and dispensers than for the needs of the patients, this prevents public accountability. By informing consumers on the quality, price, and efficiency of drugs, and strengthening their position, the pharmaceutical companies can be forced to adapt a fair business practice.

The crucial issue is, of course, awareness of consumer rights that can be mobilized to resist the unethical marketing strategies of the pharmaceuticals and drug traders. The regulatory bodies have not been able to implement the public's concerns, especially those that affect the poverty afflicted groups in Nepal. If proactive initiatives are taken to regulate the Nepali pharmaceutical market in an ethical manner, the country's health sector will grow at a reasonable rate. Without increasing the transparency and accountability in the matters of drug registration, production, promotion, distribution, prescription, and pricing, the issues of public health and consumer rights will remain marginal.

Note

1 A version of this chapter originally appeared as 'Trade in Health Service: Unfair Competition of Pharmaceutical Products in Nepal', *Dhaulagiri Journal of Sociology and Anthropology*, 3: 123–140, 2009. Used with permission.

References

Abraham, John. 2008. "Sociology of Pharmaceutical Development and Regulation: A Realist Empirical Research Programme." *Sociology of Health and Illness* 30(6): 869–885.

Abraham, John. 2010. "Pharmaceuticalization of Society in Context: Theoretical, Empirical and Health Dimensions." *Sociology* 44(4): 603–622.

GPAN. 2007. *Promotional Practices in Nepal's Pharmaceutical Market* (Unpublished Report). Kathmandu: GPAN.

Harper, Ian and Roger Jeffery. 2009. "Trust, Ethics and Spurious Medicine." *Himal South Asia* 22(8): 31–34.

Lakoff, Andrew. 2006. "High Contact: Gifts and Surveillance in Argentina." In Adriana Petryna, Andrew Lakoff and Arthur Kleinman, eds., *Global Pharmaceuticals: Ethics, Markets, Practices*, pp. 111–135. Durham: Duke University Press.

Petryna, Adriana and Arthur Kleinman. 2006. "The Pharmaceutical Nexus." In Adriana Petryna, Andrew Lakoff and Arthur Kleinman, eds., *Global Pharmaceuticals: Ethics, Markets, Practices*, pp. 1–32. Durham: Duke University Press.

Raut, Ranjan Bahadur. 2008. "Ethical Marketing of Pharmaceutical Products-Importance & Relevance in Nepalese Context." In *Souvenir of Nepal Pharma Expo 2008*, pp. 55–56. Kathmandu: APPON.

Shrestha, Umesh Lal. 2008. "Code of Conduct for Ethical Marketing in Nepal." In *Souvenir of Nepal Pharma Expo 2008*, p. 64. Kathmandu: APPON.

Subedi, Madhusudan. 2001. *Medical Anthropology of Nepal.* Kathmandu: Udaya Books.

Thapa, Bhupendra Bahadur. 2007a. "Editorial." *Drug Bulletin of Nepal* 18(2): 3–4.

Thapa, Bhupendra Bahadur. 2007b. "Editorial." *Drug Bulletin of Nepal* 19(1): 3–4.

Vaidya, Pradeep Man. 2008. "Replacing Indian Drugs Is Our Major Focus." *Business World* 55: 4–5.

Van der Geest, Sjaak. 1984. "Anthropology and Pharmaceuticals in Developing Countries." *Medical Anthropology Quarterly* 15(4): 87–90.

WHO. 2006. *Measuring Transparency in Medicines Registration, Selection and Procurement: Four Country Assessment Studies.* Geneva: WHO.

WHO. 2009. *Measuring Transparency in the Public Pharmaceutical Sector: Assessment Instrument.* Geneva: WHO.

10 Health, healing, and health care in Nepal
Current issues and an agenda for change

During the last 15 years, I have traveled in more than 60 districts, ranging from very remote mountain districts to hills, and to relatively easily accessible areas in the Tarai districts. Visiting different places and interacting with people with different cultural and economic backgrounds, and hearing their experiences, have helped me to understand the ground reality of Nepal's health system, its services and management.

This chapter gives an overview of health policies and politics in Nepal. It describes some pertinent socio-economic conditions related to health, and also offers specific suggestions for further developments within the health system. A country's development and good health among its citizens are inter-related. Thus, progress in the health sector is generally considered as a major indicator for development. This is also the case in Nepal.

A brief overview of politics and health policies in Nepal

Important political events

A country's health status is very much related to its political situation and to good governance. Nepal's political and socio-economic transformation has a long history: national unification in 1768, the autocratic Rana regime from 1846 to 1950, the establishment of a multi-party democracy in 1951, the Panchayat autocratic system (1960–1990), and the people's movement in 1990 (*Jana Aandolan* 1), led by a coalition of political parties.

Although 1990s movement generated a democratic constitution, there was widespread discontent with the constitution and with democratic reforms. The constitution did, however, create space for public criticism of the state. The Communist Party of Nepal (Maoist) was the most radical political party, and, in 1996, it presented 40 demands to the government, threatening to launch an armed struggle if the government did not take steps to address these demands. The government did not respond to these demands, and on February 12, 1996 the Maoists started a violent conflict named the 'People's War'.

Between 1996 and 2005, Nepal went through a three-polar power struggle between the King, the political parties, and the Maoist rebels. On February 1, 2005, King Gyanendra dismissed the coalition government and the elected cabinet and formed a new Council of Ministers under his own chairmanship. A second popular movement (*Jana Aandolan* 2) started in 2006, with a 12-point understanding between a Seven Parties Alliance and the Maoists. The King restored the parliament as per the demands of the popular movement. This time the people's movement, with violent demonstrations, led to King Gyanendra abdicating in 2006. The Constituent Assembly that was elected in 2008, abolished the monarchy, and started to work on a new Constitution for Nepal as a federal republic. In September 2015, the Constituent Assembly ratified the Constitution, providing a space for public criticism of government policies, prevailing social and economic inequalities, and identity-based issues in Nepal.

Health policies

The 2015 Constitution of Nepal established health as a fundamental right that would ensure quality health services to all people, including the old, the disabled, single women, the poor, the marginalized, and risk communities. Until 1975, health policy was planned and implemented *ad hoc* by ministers, secretaries, and donor organizations. The policies changed regularly, making implementation even more difficult. In 1975, the government prepared the First Long-Term Health Plan (1975–1990). The plan emphasized the provision of basic health services to a majority of the people, focusing on primary health care, hospital services, family planning, and good management. This was an honest attempt by the authorities to get things moving forward in the health field (Dixit 1999). There was, however, confusion whether to focus on individuals or on the community in order to improve the population's health status. There was also a problem with the lack of trust between health planners and health-technicians. The achievements obtained were far less than expected, the excuse being lack of budgetary recourses. The authorities argued that, in due course, results would be obtained.

An analysis of how to restructure the health services was done immediately after the people's movement in 1990. In 1991, the Ministry of

Health's National Health Policy captured the democratic essence of bringing government services closer to the people. The primary objectives of the 1991 Nepal Health Policy were to upgrade the health standards among the majority of the rural population by extending basic primary health services to the village level, and to enable people in rural areas to obtain the benefits of modern medical facilities by making such facilities accessible. The Health Policy focused on preventive, promotional, and basic primary health services, and outlined the following deficiencies in the previous health services:

- The policy, objectives, and strategies outlined for health services were not village oriented. There were deficiencies in the capability of using the available resources, the reason being that the rural plans and programs had not been formulated as per the requirements of the rural population.
- There were weaknesses in the implementation of plans and programs.
- The supervision, monitoring, and evaluation of the programs were not conducted in a regular manner.
- The resources were centralized.
- The posts approved for district level health institutions and organizations were not filled.

The main elements in the preventive health services were these: providing family planning, safe motherhood, and maternal child health; expanded immunization; controlling diarrhea, acute respiratory infections, tuberculosis, leprosy, malaria, kalazar, and communicable diseases; initiating means to prevent non-communicable diseases; introducing primary health services in urban slums; and the prevention and control of AIDS.

The promotional health services focused on health education and information, nutrition, and environmental health. It was assumed that one of the main reasons for the low health standard among people was the lack of public awareness of health matters and health education, and that information went from institutions in Kathmandu and other urban centers to rural areas. To improve the nutritional status among children the programs prioritized the promotion of breast-feeding, growth monitoring, preventing disorders due to deficiency of iodine, iron, and vitamin A, and health education to enable mothers to meet the children's daily needs through locally available resources. The environmental health program focused, through various media, on personal hygiene, solid waste management, and the construction of toilets.

The curative health services focused on establishing one sub-health post or health post at the Village Development Committee level, and primary health care centers at the election constituency level. These sub-health posts and health posts would provide immunization, family planning, maternal and child health education, nutrition, and treatment of malaria, leprosy, and tuberculosis. There should also be at least one hospital in each district that could provide outdoor and indoor services, family planning, maternity and child health services, immunization, and emergency services. The National Health Policy recommended that there be established one hospital in each zone, one hospital in each development region, and well-equipped centrally located hospitals with sophisticated diagnostic and other facilities.

The 1991 National Health Policy focused on the importance of technically competent human resources at all the health facilities, and to provide training centers and academic institutions. The policy also promoted the involvement of the private sector by providing conditions that might encourage such investments in health care services.

This health policy led to the introduction of many new sub-sectoral health policies like the National Blood Policy (1993), the National Drug Policy (1995), the National Mental Health Policy (1995), the National Ayurveda Health Policy (1996), the National Safe Motherhood Policy (1998), and the National AIDS Policy (1995).

During the interaction with various stakeholders, ranging from government representatives to people in nongovernmental organizations, and academicians in both urban and rural areas, I was told that the government health policy mainly addressed issues in rural areas, saying little about the health needs of the urban poor. The policy called for upgrading the health standards among a majority of the rural population, but it gave little attention to access to, and use of, health services by women, children, and by the poor and excluded people. The policy did not deal with intersectoral issues such as water, sanitation, medical waste management, climate change, environmental health, and geriatric services. It also did not spell out issues related to social security and social health protection.

The Second Long-Term Health Plan (1997–2017) came in 1997 (MoH 1999). This 20-year perspective plan called for the following:

• Improving the health status particularly of those whose health needs are often not met: vulnerable people, women and children, people living in rural areas, the poor, under-privileged, and marginalized people.
• Extending essential health care services at all public health facilities.

- Developing an appropriate number of technically competent and socially responsible health personnel, particularly in rural areas.
- Improving the management and organization of the public health sector.
- Developing appropriate roles for NGOs, and for public and private sector participation in providing health care.
- Improving inter- and intra-sector coordination, and supporting the effective decentralization of health care services with full community participation.

In 2004, the Government of Nepal introduced a 'Health Sector Strategy: An Agenda for Reform' (MoH 2004). Its purpose was to improve aid effectiveness by coordinating the efforts of national and foreign development partners into a single program that was owned and led by the government (HMG-N and NPC 2002). Such a program could put the country on the track to achieve the 2015 Millennium Development Goals for health.

After the popular movement in April 2006, access to health care services was declared a fundamental human right, and people's expectation towards health care grew significantly. The 2007 Interim Constitution, for the first time in Nepal's history, enshrined the state's commitment to its citizens' health.

The 1991 National Health Policy was not adequate to ensure each citizen's fundamental right to health, and to manage the various problems and challenges. The 2014 National Health Policy (GoN and MoHP 2071BS) had the following guiding principles:

- To ensure the citizens' fundamental right to quality health services.
- To ensure the citizens' right to information regarding health services.
- Programs must be formulated and implemented on the basis of equity and social justice to ensure that the poor, marginalized groups, and risk communities have access to public health services.
- Citizens from all walks of life should be inspired to take advantage of the health services.
- Policies and programs pertaining to the promotion, protection, and rehabilitation of citizens should be included in the state's policies for other sectors.
- The private sector should be encouraged to participate in such a way that citizens easily can access affordable quality health services.
- Means and resources received from national and international agencies should be mobilized in such a way that health policy and programs can be implemented efficiently.

- All the health services provided by government or nongovernmental institutions and organizations should be regulated and monitored.
- Health service delivery should be made accountable.

The National Health Policy, formulated in 2014, envisioned that all Nepali citizens should have physical, mental, social, and spiritual health that could lead to productive and quality lives. Available resources should be used optimally by fostering a strategic cooperation between health service providers, service users, and other stakeholders. The goal of this policy was to provide health services to every citizen through an equitable and accountable health system. The objectives of the policy were the following:

- To provide the basic health services free of cost.
- To establish effective, accountable, and accessible health facilities equipped with essential drugs, diagnostics, and skilled human resources.
- To promote people's participation and sense of ownership in health services provision.
- To promote the involvement of the private sector and nongovernmental organizations in providing health services effectively, in collaboration with the government.

The 2014 National Health Policy presented a forward-looking agenda for improving the health and wellbeing of all citizens of Nepal. It articulated the nation's commitment towards achieving universal health care coverage. It aimed at putting health as a central component of the overall development, to build partnerships and establish multi-sector collaboration. The policy recognized the importance of creating a healthy environment and to encourage people, especially the young, to choose a healthy lifestyle. It also had an inclusive approach to Ayurveda and other traditional medical systems.

The constitutional provisions

The 2007 Interim Constitution established the right of all Nepali citizens to free basic health services, the right to a clean environment, access to education and means for a fair livelihood within a social environment free of discrimination and institutionalized inequality.

On September 22, 2015, the Constituent Assembly ratified the new Constitution. Its Article 35 stated: "Every citizen shall have the right to seek basic health care services from the state and no citizen shall be deprived of emergency health care." It also stated that:

> each person shall have the right to be informed about his/her health condition with regard to health care services, each person shall have equal access to health care and each citizen shall have the right to access to clean water and hygiene.

The Constitution included five more rights:

Box 10.1

Article 38. Right of Women: Every woman shall have the right relating to safe motherhood and reproductive health (Article 38(2)).

Article 39. Right of Children: Every child shall have the right to education, health care nurturing, appropriate upbringing, sports, recreation, and overall personality development, provided either by its family or by the State (Article 39(2)).

Article 40. Right of Dalits: In order to provide health care and social security to the Dalit community, special arrangements shall be made in accordance with law (Article 40(3)).

Article 42: Right to Social Justice: Citizens who are economically very poor and communities on the verge of extinction, shall have the right to special opportunities and facilities regarding education, health, housing, employment, food and social security, to ensure their protection, progress, empowerment and development (Article 42(2)).

People with physical impairments shall have the right to a dignified way of life, to equal access to social services and facilities, and to keep their specific identity (Article 42(3)).

Article 51. State Policies: The State shall gradually increase necessary investments in the public health sector in order to make the citizens healthy (Article 51 (h) (5)).

Measures shall be taken to ensure easily available and equal access to high quality health care for all (Article 51 (h) (6)).

The current situation

Over the last 50 years, the conditions within the health sector have improved considerably. After the introduction of a multi-party system in Nepal in 1990, notable progress has been made in improving the primary health care services throughout the country by establishing primary health care facilities at the electoral constituency level and health posts at the VDC level. Also outreach services have improved, providing female MCHW, VHW, and female community health workers at the VDC level. Through successive five years plans various governments in Nepal have made an effort to improve people's health conditions and enhance their access to basic health care.

Safe water and sanitation

The basic determinants for better health are still in a critical state in Nepal. Poor access to drinking water, sanitation facilities, and poor hygiene, are causing skin diseases, ARI, and diarrheal diseases, all leading preventable diseases. The 2015 Constitution of Nepal stated that access to water is a fundamental right, and the Thirteenth Three Year Plan included a goal to achieve universal access to basic drinking water by 2017.

According to the National 2011 Census, nearly 85 percent of all households get drinking water from a well or through pipes. Some households are still using water from rivers and streams, but this water is relatively unsafe to drink. Households in urban areas have greater access to improved sources for drinking water than households in rural areas.

Use of improved toilet facilities prevent people from coming into contact with human waste and helps to reduce the transmission of communicable diseases such as cholera and typhoid. According to the 2016 NDHS, only 62 percent of the households had good toilet facilities, which clearly shows that people still use a bush or the open field for defecation. There has been substantial improvements in the use of better sanitation facilities. Households using improved facilities almost doubled from 38 percent in 2011 to 62 percent in 2016. Similarly, the percentage of households with no toilet facilities decreased from 36 percent to 15 percent (Ministry of Health, Nepal; New ERA; and ICF 2017). Hand washing provides protection against communicable diseases, and is promoted by the Government of Nepal. The 2016 NDHS data showed that soap and water for hand washing were available among only 47 percent, while 20 percent did not have water, soap, or any other cleansing agents in place for hand washing. Similarly, 39 percent of the households in the lowest wealth quintile did not have water or any other cleansing agents for hand washing (Ministry of Health, Nepal; New ERA; and ICF 2017).

Food

The 2011 NDHS showed that only 49 percent of all households in Nepal were food secure and had access to food throughout the year. Urban households were more food secure (67 percent) than rural households (46 percent). The proportion of food secure households was higher in the Tarai (52 percent) than in the hills (47 percent) and in the mountain regions (41 percent). The 10 percent most wealthy households were much more likely to be food secure (82 percent) than the least wealthy households (18 percent) (Ministry of Health and Population, New ERA, and ICF International Inc. 2012).

The food secure households have more or less remained constant from 2011 to 2016 (49 percent in 2011 versus 48 percent in 2016). Urban households are more likely (54 percent) to be food secure than rural households (39 percent). A large proportion of households in Province 6 (42 percent) and the lowest wealth quintile (39 percent) fall in the moderately food insecure category. Similarly, the highest proportions of severely food insecure households are in the lowest wealth quintile (22 percent) and in Province 6 (18 percent) (Ministry of Health, Nepal; New ERA; and ICF 2017).

Cooking fuel sources

Nepalese households depend heavily on traditional energy sources for cooking. Firewood is the main source of cooking fuel in rural areas, followed by kerosene and LP Gas. LP gas has been the more popular energy source in urban areas whereas firewood, cow-dung, and agricultural residues are widely used as an energy source in the rural areas, the latter types producing indoor pollution that lead to health problems such as acute respiratory diseases, especially among women and children.

Life expectancy at birth

Life expectancy at birth for both males and females has been increasing gradually from 1954 to 2011. In 1954, life expectancy at birth was 27.1 years for males, 28.5 years for females. These figures increased to 60.2 for males, 60.8 years for females in 2000, and to 67.7 for males, 70.8 for females in 2015. Such a significant change in life expectancy at birth is due to more modern health facilities that have reduced the death rates, especially infant and child mortality.

Mortality

In response to the International Conference on Population and Development in 1994, Nepal endorsed a Reproductive Health Research Strategy in 1998 (Family Health Division, MoH 1998). This document identified an integrated reproductive health package for Nepal, including safe motherhood as one of its key components. Following the Reproductive Health Research Strategy, the National Safe Motherhood Plan (2002–2017) was developed in 2002 (Family Health Division, MoH 2002).

The 2016 NDHS showed that neonatal mortality rate was 21 deaths per 1,000 live births, while the under-five mortality rate was 39 deaths per 1,000 live births. Between 1996 and 2016, neonatal mortality fell from 50 to 21 deaths per 1,000 live births, infant mortality declined from 78 to 32 deaths per 1,000 live births, and under-five mortality fell from 118 to 39 deaths per 1,000 live births. There are large variations by province in childhood mortality. For example, neonatal mortality ranges from a low of 15 deaths per 1,000 live births in Province 4 to a high of 41 in Province 7 (Ministry of Health, Nepal; New ERA; and ICF 2017)

Institutional delivery

Nepal is promoting safe motherhood through initiatives such as providing free delivery care and transportation incentive schemes to women delivering in a health facility. Subsidies are also provided to health facilities for free delivery care on the basis of deliveries conducted (Ministry of Health, Nepal; New ERA; and ICF 2017). Increasing the percentage of births delivered in health facilities is important for reducing deaths due to complications during pregnancy.

There was a minimal increase in institutional deliveries from 1996 to 2001. However, the proportion doubled to 18 percent in 2006 and doubled again with 35 percent in 2011. Between 2011 and 2016 there was a remarkable increase (57 percent) in the proportion of institutional deliveries. Delivery in a health facility varies widely by ecological region. The proportion of deliveries in health facilities is higher among births to mothers with an SLC and higher education (85 percent) than among births to mothers without any education (36 percent). A similar pattern is seen in terms of wealth: delivery at a health facility is significantly lower among births among the 34 percent least wealthy than among the 90 percent most wealthy people (Ministry of Health, Nepal; New ERA; and ICF 2017).

Health workforce

The 2010 WHO Report listed Nepal among the 59 countries with a critical shortage of human resources in the health sector. The existing situation presents a mixed scenario with plenty of equipment that is not used efficiently. The reason is a top-down decision-making process that prevails despite the fact that policy amendments have emphasized the empowerment of local government to regulate and monitor the local development agencies. There is high concentration of health workers in urban areas and marked geographical unequal distribution of all types of health workers.

Mismanagement in selecting appropriate candidates for in-service training has resulted in repetition and oversight. As a result, some health workers without political and social links to a higher authority have been frustrated. Another reason for the frustration was that the health workers were transferred based on political connections rather than on a human resource policy that took into account qualifications and performances. Also the security issue affected the health workers' motivation to stay in some places.

Urban-rural differences

Despite the improvements described in the earlier sections, the health status and health services available to people in rural Nepal are among the worst in the modern world (Woollard 2005). Health services have not reached the citizens in all regions and within all social classes, malnutrition is observed among nearly half of the children under five and among women of reproductive age, and non-communicable diseases as well as psychiatric illnesses and dental problems are increasing every day. Almost 50 percent of Nepali doctors, most sophisticated and large private nursing homes and hospitals, trained medical professionals, and health facilities, are concentrated in the Kathmandu Valley. (Dixit 1999; Streefland 1985; Justice 1986; Subedi 1989; Subedi 2001a). Also health related policymaking and decisions regarding the allocation of resources are done in Kathmandu.

There certainly is a shortage of resources, but health care services are also unequally distributed. The limited facilities available are concentrated in the urban areas, including hospitals and medical colleges with diagnostic and surgical equipment similar to that found in developed countries. They swallow up a very high proportion of available funds, leaving little to support the simple health posts and sub-health posts and clinics needed by the urban and rural poor. Thus, existing political and legal systems protect conditions that favor the urban elite (Shrestha 1998). Health is more accessible and cheaper for those who are in the golden circle of the 'haves' than among the 'have-nots'.

Health care centers are frequently lacking in trained personnel and medical supplies, and a large segment of the population relies on traditional healers. Children are particularly vulnerable, because they are less likely to be brought long distances to health centers and they are more prone to diseases than adults.

The private sector

There is a considerable private sector in the delivery of health care in Nepal. Many curative institutions, pharmaceutical factories, and medical equipment industries are privately owned, making profit-making an important factor for health care delivery as well as for the production and sale of drugs and materials. The consequence is that, broadly speaking, the best services and facilities are available in those places where wealthy people are living and wealth is concentrated (Streefland 1985; Subedi 2001a).

The consequence of the urban-biased health system described is an increased call for privatization. Nepal's health plans clearly show a liberal, open, and competitive policy in which the Government of Nepal provides opportunities for multinational pharmaceutical companies and bilateral companies in favor of private health services (Harper 2002). The state's responsibility to provide an adequate health sector is being reduced in the name of competition and the free market. For the periphery it means low quality health care services and relatively low numbers of drug sellers and medical practitioners. Besides, the overall lack of qualified doctors, partly as a consequence of the brain drain, and the large demand for curative services, in combination with the state's control of the periphery, create an excellent environment for the activities of unqualified medical practitioners and unlicensed drug sellers (Subedi 2001b).

Obviously there are variations in this pattern, largely coinciding with regional differences in poverty. Private investments in the health sector have not been in programs aimed at taking care of particular health needs or to deliver adequate health care services to people in general. There are also great regional differences in the private sector's involvement, particularly between the Tarai and the mountain areas. In the Tarai, doctors and pharmacies are located in the urban centers, and only unqualified practitioners and drug sellers in the villages; the farther away from a town and the less populated an area is, the lower the quality of the services provided (Karkee 2002; Subedi 2001a). In the hills, pharmacies and doctors are primarily found in the Kathmandu Valley and in the regional administrative and commercial centers.

Current challenges

Although the health sector has already achieved notable progress and the country is moving in a positive direction, there are still many problems and challenges within and outside the health sector. The 2014 National Health Policy listed the following major challenges:

- The health services have not reached the citizens in every region, social class, and community as envisioned in the constitution.
- Despite continuous efforts by the state, obesity is growing in the urban areas, and malnutrition is observed among nearly half of the children under five and among women of reproductive age.
- Health related problems are increasing because of climate change, increasing food insecurity and natural calamities.
- Non-communicable diseases such as cancer, heart diseases, high blood pressure, diabetics, kidney diseases, liver and lung diseases as well as psychiatric illnesses and dental problems, are increasing. Likewise, the number of people dying because of accidents and injury is increasing.
- Despite its importance, the state has not been able to adequately prioritize health among the urban poor and in marginalized communities, neither has it prioritized geriatric health, mental health, genetic diseases, environmental health, occupational health, sexual and reproductive health, adolescent health, and youth programs.

Health care cannot remain neutral and be limited to bodily maladies; so much of what influences good health is situated in the society (Mikesell 2003). In spite of the general increase in the number of health facilities in the country, one of the most serious concerns of any society is the existence of large segments of the population who are denied adequate or any attention to their health. They are individuals or groups who, for a variety of political, social, and economic reasons, are consciously or unconsciously discriminated against, and who receive less attention than the majority of the population. Commercialization of education and health has affected the lives and wellbeing of a majority of the people who live in both urban and rural areas. Without health science institutions that can identify and address major health concerns among the poor people, health for all is a dream. As most of the medical schools are private, profit-oriented institutions, high tuition fees do not encourage young people in poorer areas to apply. Voices in rural and disadvantaged communities are not easily heard, and patients with serious diseases suffer.

Some agendas for change

The end in 2006 of the ten-year-long armed conflict marked the beginning of a new era of peace and cooperation. The agreement reached in 2006 between the Government of Nepal and the Communist Party of Nepal (Maoist) stated that the Constituent Assembly would work for progressive political solutions, democratic restructuring of the state, and social, economic, and cultural transformations of the Nepalese society. They also agreed to prepare a common development concept that would facilitate a socio-economic transformation of the country and also to ensure economic prosperity in a not-too-distant future. Both parties committed themselves to respect and guarantee the people's right to food security and good health. The agreement also ascertained that there would not be any political interference in the production and utilization of food, and its transportation and distribution. To meet people's health needs, a concrete health policy and programs should be developed.

Despite progress in people's health conditions, significant equity gaps persist. Many citizens still face economic, social, geographic, and cultural barriers. There also are problems related to political and administrative malfunctioning.

Economic factors

Economic factors play a crucial role for the conditions within the health sector in Nepal, affecting the distribution of health facilities and medical equipment, and also the health status of different socio-economic groups and their access to health services. For instance, the 2011 NDHS showed the bitter fact that the under-five mortality rate in the poorest income groups was twice as much as in the richest one, and some 10 percent of the children did not receive full immunization.

Nepal is committed to expand universal health coverage to ensure the whole population access to equity health services. This can be done by providing basic health services free-of-charge, and by providing other services beyond the basic health package at an affordable cost through targeted subsidies and various social health protection schemes. People should, for instance, be compensated for the loss of income while seeking health care.

To identify those families, social groups, and communities that are excluded or underserved, and the reasons for this exclusion, is a fundamental precondition for improving their health coverage. It is important to note that barriers associated with being poor and excluded (and female) exist across all socio-economic groups, and that a simple distinction between castes or ethnic groups is inadequate as a basis for planning and delivering health services. At the same time, ignoring caste and ethnicity can lead to an ineffective service delivery.

The private sector

Currently there is a tendency toward marked expansion in the private sector in urban areas, characterized by high cost for health care, the pull of scarce human talent from the less remunerative government sector, expensive medical procedures, excessive laboratory studies, and the coexistence of clandestine private practice under the cover of public health care institutions. The subtle connections between the two need careful analysis. Also the social and economic impact of unrestrained use of technology for treating individual patients needs to be studied. The current vertical program between the various divisions in the Department of Health Services and among the nongovernmental organizations should be integrated with the general health services, with a view to their ultimate transfer to the public health services.

Decentralization

The most fundamental and challenging feature of the HEALTH FOR ALL framework in Nepal is the strong commitment to decentralization. This will help democratize the system by returning decision making to the local level, and increase transparency and accountability. This can be done by increased involvement by local groups, such as mothers groups, community forest user groups, and local self-help groups. This can empower the women, and promote supportive cultural practices and healthy lifestyles within their communities.

While there is a clear structure for health administration in Nepal, it is not functioning efficiently and, therefore, it is undermining confidence in the government's capacity to provide basic services in an equitable manner. This requires more systematic and regular mapping of facilities at the local level throughout the country, and the extent to which different social groups use these facilities. For instance, lack of privacy keeps many women away from government facilities, and Dalits and poor people feel they are treated in a disrespectful and discriminatory way. Access to the government health facilities is partly hindered by short and unreliable opening hours, and that health care workers often are absent from the health facility.

Even with good plans, implementing them seem to be deeply rooted in endemic factors within the health system, such as patronage in appointments, and inequalities in the way that resources are clustered near the main towns, and that they, therefore, do not reach the poorest areas.

Technology

Nepal's occasional natural disasters and climate change affect also people's health. Technology can help to treat some of these problems. However, the bulk of the health problems in Nepal stems from the inability to apply fully the basic or classical health technologies for providing safe drinking water, environmentally appropriate sanitation, immunization, food safety, and nutritious food. Today, Nepal can use the very same techniques that were instrumental for obtaining the great changes in people's health in other parts of the world during the first industrial revolution.

Administrative and political factors

The political leadership and health administrators have sought to secure an aura of social legitimacy for their actions by pointing to some not very relevant social, cultural, and psychological issues raised by social scientists. Value laden issues such as modernization versus traditionalism, and urban culture versus traditional rural folk culture, have been used to justify the urban and privileged class biased health services in Nepal. Maybe the 2015 Constitution of Nepal can lead to a change; it established the right of all Nepali citizens to free basic health services, the right to a clean environment, and access to education and to the means to a secure livelihood in a social environment free of discrimination and institutionalized inequality.

Nepal's new federal structure requires changes also in the health sector. Special emphasis should be given on decentralization and to strengthen local health facilities and their governance. The Ministry of Health and its subordinate authorities must be restructured to make them more responsive to current health needs.

Conclusion

Now is a moment of historic opportunity. With effective leadership, well-managed coordinated programs, appropriate health delivery systems, with a judicious mix of the classical time-honored and newer technologies, and professional as well as social commitment, the health conditions of the Nepali people can be improved rapidly even within the contexts of limited resources and slow economic growth. Such a strategy is consistent with the view that health cannot be advanced without a simultaneous and sustained social development in general.

Those committed to identify themselves with the interest of the poor (health workers, political activists, scholars, voluntary agencies, media persons, and others) must play a very active role in the fight against the forces which stand in the way of the implementation of good health for all. Those committed to the poor must stand squarely on the side of the poor. Their struggle should be against the creation of dependency particularly on foreign agencies for supplies, and against the nefarious move to sell such obviously defective and often harmful programs through manipulating people with the weapons of social marketing. They also must play a positive role in demonstrating that there can be an alternative system which, with the same resources, much better can serve the poor by focusing on people's own needs, developing people-oriented technologies, and building an organization to deliver such technologies.

Nepal faces several health related problems. While communicable diseases continue to pose problems, there is now a growing prevalence of non-communicable diseases. There are also increasing threats of natural disasters due to climate change, and there are an increasing number of deaths and injuries due to road accidents, violence, and injuries. Many citizens continue to face financial, socio-cultural, geographical, and institutional barriers in accessing health services. Despite efforts to reduce gender inequality, women in Nepal are still marginalized, and this affects their health and wellbeing. Increasing access to health care services and improving the quality of health care remain a major challenge. Due to the rapid urbanization, the expansion of urban health services is a burning challenge. Regional and international cooperation in health service development must be based on a solid foundation of indigenous public health.

Political interests and interference have been prevalent also within the health sector. The prime mover for action to improve the situation must come from within the country. One example is Dr Govinda KC, a senior professor and orthopedic surgeon at Tribhuvan University. His non-violent movement, with several fasts-unto-death in 2015, 2016, and 2017, was aimed at improving the medical education in Nepal and to get rid of the country's so called medical mafia. Dr KC dedicated his services and income to the poor, the marginalized, and the underserved population in Nepal as well as in other countries, to make his opponents change their understanding and sense of values. The government agreed with most of his demands, but due to political pressure from the political parties and from the unregulated private sector, the state has not been able to implement these genuine demands. To improve the health services and the quality of health care in Nepal, the active participation of the citizens and a transparent and ethical public and private sector, and of nongovernmental organizations, are necessary.

Overcoming existing health inequalities requires a sustained multi-prolonged strategy to address barriers against both demand and supply, and to build the capacity of the Ministry of Health to lead this agenda. Improvements within the health sector require efforts across several sectors. Thus, health becomes part of the broader agenda for developing the country in general.

The 2015 Constitution of Nepal, the 2014 National Health Policy, and the periodic plans of the National Planning Commission (NPC), recognize that women, Dalits, people living with disabilities, sexual and gender minorities, and people in geographically remote areas, experience barriers against benefitting from the nation's development. This warrants a major thrust with affirmative action to ensure that the citizens have greater access to health services.

References

Dixit, Hemang. 1999. *The Quest for Health*. Kathmandu: Educational Enterprise (P) Ltd.

Family Health Division, MoH. 1998. *National Reproductive Health Research Strategy*. Kathmandu: Family Health Division, Ministry of Health.

Family Health Division, MoH. 2002. *National Safe Motherhood Plan (2002-2017)*. Kathmandu: Family Health Division, Ministry of Health.

GoN and MoHP. 2071BS. *Rastriya Swastha Niti 2071 [National Health Policy 2014]*. Kathmandu: Government of Nepal, Ministry of Health and Population.

Harper, Ian. 2002. "Capsular Promise as Public Health: A Critique of the Nepal National Vitamin A Program." *Studies in Nepali History and Society* 7(1): 137–173.

HMG-N and NPC. 2002. *Tenth Plan (2002–2007)*. Kathmandu: His Majesty's Government, National Planning Commission.

Justice, Judith. 1986. *Policies, Plans, and People: Foreign Aid and Health Development*. Berkeley: University of California Press.

Karkee, Shiba Bahadur. 2002. *Issues in Antibacterial Provision in Primary Health Care in Nepal.* Unpublished Thesis, The Royal Danish School of Pharmacy, Department of Social Pharmacy, Denmark.

Mikesell, Stephen. 2003. "Editorial." *Journal of Physicians for Social Responsibility, Nepal* 4(1).

Ministry of Health. 1991. *National Health Policy 1991.* Kathmandu: Planning, Monitoring and Supervision Division.

Ministry of Health. 1997. *Second Long-Term Health Plan 1997–2017.* Kathmandu: Health Sector Reform Unit.

Ministry of Health and Population, New ERA, and ICF International Inc. 2012. *Nepal Demographic and Health Survey 2011.* Kathmandu: Ministry of Health and Population, New ERA, and Macro International Inc.

Ministry of Health, Nepal; New ERA; and ICF. 2017. *Nepal Demographic and Health Survey 2016.* Kathmandu: Ministry of Health, Nepal.

MoH. 1999. *Second Long-Term Health Plan.* Kathmandu: Ministry of Health.

MoH. 2004. *Vulnerable Community Development Plan for Nepal Health Sector Program Implementation Plan.* Kathmandu: Health Sector Reform Unit, Planning Division, Ministry of Health.

Shrestha, Mathura Prasad. 1998. "What I Believe about ENHR." *Sachetana, Journal of Essential National Health Research Nepal* 1(1). Kathmandu: Nepal Health Research Council (NHRC).

Streefland, Pieter. 1985. "The Frontier of Modern Western Medicine in Nepal." *Social Science and Medicine* 20(11): 1151–1159.

Subedi, Janardan. 1989. "Modern Health Services and Health Care Behavior: A Survey in Kathmandu, Nepal." *Journal of Health and Social Behavior* 30: 412–420.

Subedi, Madhusudan Sharma. 2001a. "Development and Underdevelopment of Modern Health Services in Nepal." *Deva Vani* 4(4). Kathmandu: Devaghat Vedic Adhyatmic Parishad.

Subedi, Madhusudan Sharma. 2001b. *Medical Anthropology of Nepal.* Kathmandu: Udaya Books.

Woollard, Robert. 2005. *Feasibility Study for the Proposed Patan University of Health Sciences.* A Report Submitted to the Medical School Steering Committee/Task Force. Kathmandu: Unpublished Report.

Index